MOLECULAR PATHOGENESIS OF PANCREATIC CANCER

Biomedical and Health Research

Volume 41

Earlier published in this series

Vol. 10. F.F. Cruz-Sánchez, R. Ravid and M.L. Cuzner (Eds.), Neuropathological Diagnostic Criteria for Brain Banking
Vol. 11. S.S. Baig (Ed.), Cancer Research at the European Level
Vol. 12. M. Maio (Ed.), Immunology of Human Melanoma
Vol. 13. V.K. Hopsu-Havu, M. Järvinen and H. Kirschke (Eds.), Proteolysis in Cell Functions
Vol. 14. G. ter Heege (Ed.), EURO-QUAL
Vol. 15. N. Katunuma, H. Kido, H. Fritz and J. Travis (Eds.), Medical Aspects of Proteases and Protease Inhibitors
Vol. 16. P.I. Haris and D. Chapman (Eds.), New Biomedical Materials
Vol. 17. J.J.F. Schroots, R. Fernandez-Ballesteros and G. Rudinger (Eds.), Aging in Europe
Vol. 18. R. Leidl (Ed.), Health Care and its Financing in the Single European Market
Vol. 19. P. Jenner and R. Demirdamar (Eds.), Dopamine Receptor Subtypes
Vol. 20. P.I. Haris and D. Chapman (Eds.), Biomembrane Structures
Vol. 21. N. Yoganandan, F.A. Pintar, S.J. Larson and A. Sances Jr. (Eds.), Frontiers in Head and Neck Trauma
Vol. 22. J. Matsoukas and T. Mavromoustakos (Eds.), Bioactive Peptides in Drug Discovery and Design: Medical Aspects
Vol. 23. M. Hallen (Ed.), Human Genome Analysis
Vol. 24. S.S. Baig (Ed.), Cancer Research Supported under BIOMED 1
Vol. 25. N.J. Gooderham (Ed.), Drug Metabolism: Towards the Next Millennium
Vol. 26. P. Jenner (Ed.), A Molecular Biology Approach to Parkinson's Disease
Vol. 27. P.A. Frey and D.B. Northrop (Eds.), Enzymatic Mechanisms
Vol. 28. A.M.N. Gardner and R. Fox, The Venous System in Health and Disase
Vol. 29. G. Pawelec (Ed.), EUCAMBIS: Immunology and Ageing in Europe
Vol. 30. J.F. Stoltz, M. Singh and P. Riha, Hemorheology in Practice
Vol. 31. B.J. Njio, A. Stenvik, R.S. Ireland and B. Prahl-Andersen (Eds.), EURO-QUAL
Vol. 32. In production
Vol. 33. H.H. Goebel, S.E. Mole and B.D. Lake (Eds.), The Neuronal Ceroid Lipofuscinoses (Batten Disease)
Vol. 34. G.J. Bellingan and G.J. Laurent (Eds.), Acute Lung Injury: From Inflammation to Repair
Vol. 35. M. Schlaud (Ed.), Comparison and Harmonisation of Denominator Data for Primary Health Care Research in Countries of the European Community
Vol. 36. F.F. Parl, Estrogens, Estrogen Receptor and Breast Cancer
Vol. 37. J.M. Ntambi (Ed.), Adipocyte Biology and Hormone Signaling
Vol. 38. N. Yoganandan and F.A. Pintar (Eds.), Frontiers in Whiplash Trauma
Vol. 39. J.-M. Graf von der Schulenburg (Ed.), The Influence of Economic Evaluation Studies on Health Care Decision-Making
Vol. 40. H. Leino-Kilpi, M. Välimäki, M. Arndt, T. Dassen, M. Gasull, C. Lemonidou, P.A. Scott, G. Bansemir, E. Cabrera, H. Papaevangelou and J. Mc Parland, Patient's Autonomy, Privacy and Informed Consent

ISSN: 0929-6743

Molecular Pathogenesis of Pancreatic Cancer

Edited by

T.M. Gress

Department of Internal Medicine, Universitätsklinikum Ulm, Ulm, Germany

IOS Press

Ohmsha

Amsterdam • Berlin • Oxford • Tokyo • Washington, DC

ISBN 1 58603 040 X (IOS Press)
ISBN 4 274 90374 5 C3047 (Ohmsha)
Library of Congress Catalog Card Number: 00-103712

Publisher
IOS Press
Nieuwe Hemweg 6B
1013 BG Amsterdam
The Netherlands
fax: +31 20 620 3419
e-mail: order@iospress.nl

Distributor in the UK and Ireland
IOS Press/Lavis Marketing
73 Lime Walk
Headington
Oxford OX3 7AD
England
fax: +44 1865 75 0079

Distributor in the USA and Canada
IOS Press, Inc.
5795-G Burke Centre Parkway
Burke, VA 22015
USA
fax: +1 703 323 3668
e-mail: iosbooks@iospress.com

Distributor in Germany
IOS Press
Spandauer Strasse 2
D-10178 Berlin
Germany
fax: +49 30 242 3113

Distributor in Japan
Ohmsha, Ltd.
3-1 Kanda Nishiki-cho
Chiyoda-ku, Tokyo 101
Japan
fax: +81 3 3233 2426

PRINTED IN THE NETHERLANDS

Members of the Concerted Action:

1. Project Coordinator:
   PD Dr. Thomas Gress
   Universitätsklinikum Ulm
   Abt. Innere Medizin I
   Robert-Koch-Str. 8
   D – 89081 Ulm

2. Dr. Hans Lehrach
   Max-Planck-Institut für Molekulare Genetik
   Ihnestr. 73
   D - 14194 Berlin (Dahlem)

3. Dr. Jörg Hoheisel
   Deutsches Krebsforschungszentrum (DKFZ)
   Im Neuenheimer Feld 506
   D - 69120 Heidelberg

4. Prof. Nicholas Lemoine
   ICRF Molecular Oncology Unit
   Imperial College of Science, Technology & Medicine
   Hammersmith Campus
   GB - London W12 ONN

5. Dr. Fransisco Real
   Institut Municipal d'Investigació Mèdica, IMIM
   Department of Immunology
   Calle Doctor Aiguader, 80
   ES - 08003 Barcelona

6. Prof. Aldo Scarpa
   Università di Verona
   Istituto di Anatomia Patologica
   Strada Le Grazie, 8
   I - 37134 Verona

7. Prof. Dr. W. Schmiegel
   Medizinische Klinik der Ruhr-Universität
   Knappschaftskrankenhaus Langendreer
   In der Schornau 23-25
   D - 44892 Bochum

8. Dr. Martine Muleris
   Institut Curie
   26, Rue d'Ulm
   F - 75248 Paris Cedex 05

9. Dr. Gabor Varga
   Hungarian Academy of Sciences
   Institute of Experimental Medicine
   P.O. Box 67
   H – 1450 Budapest

Participants and contributors

ADELL, Teresa	Unitat de Biologia Cellular i Molecular, Institut Municipal d'Investigació Mèdica, Doctor Aiguader, 80, E-08003 Barcelona, Spain. Tel.: (+34) 93 221 1009, Fax: (+34) 93 221 3237
AMILLET, Jean-Michel	UMR 147 CNRS, Institut Curie, 26 rue d'Ulm, 75248 Paris Cedex 05, France. Tel: (+33) 1 42 34 66 75, Fax: (+33) 1 42 34 66 74
BOECK, Wolfgang	Abteilung Innere Medizin I, Universitätsklinikum Ulm, Robert Koch Str. 8, D-89081 Ulm, Germany Tel.: (+49) 731 502 4311/4312, Fax: (+49) 731 502 4302.
BURGHARDT, Beata	Institute of Experimental Medicine, Hungarian Academy of Sciences, H-1083 Budapest, Hungary. Tel: (+36) 1 210 0819, ext. 133, Fax: (+36) 1 210 0813 E-mail: burghard@koki.hu
CZINK, Claudia	Functional Genome Analysis, German Cancer Research Center, Im Neuenheimer Feld 506, Room 20, D-69120 Heidelberg, Germany. Tel: (+49) 622 142 4683, Fax: (+49) 622 142 4682
CRNOGORAC-JURCEVIC, Tatjana	ICRF Molecular Oncology Unit, Dept of Cancer Medicine, Imperial College School of Medicine, Hammersmith Campus, Du Cane Road. London W12 0NN, UK. Tel: (+44) 181 383 3975, Fax: (+44) 181 383 3258

DIEHL, Frank	Functional Genome Analysis, German Cancer Research Center, Im Neuenheimer Feld 506, Room 20, D-69120 Heidelberg, Germany. Tel: (+49) 622 142 4683, Fax: (+49) 622 142 4682
GOMÈZ-CUADRADO, Alicia	Unitat de Biologia Cellular i Molecular, Institut Municipal d'Investigació Mèdica, Doctor Aiguader, 80, E-08003 Barcelona, Spain. Tel.: (+34) 93 221 1009, Fax: (+34) 93 221 3237
FROHME, Marcus	Functional Genome Analysis, German Cancer Research Center, Im Neuenheimer Feld 506, Room 20, D-69120 Heidelberg, Germany. Tel: (+49) 622 142 4683, Fax: (+49) 622 142 4682
GOUBIN, Gerard	UMR 147 CNRS, Institut Curie, 26 rue d'Ulm, F-75248 Paris Cedex 05, France. Tel: (+33) 1 42 34 66 75, Fax: (+33) 1 42 34 66 74
GRESS, Thomas	Abteilung Innere Medizin I, Universitätsklinukum, Robert Koch Str. 8, D-89081 Ulm, Germany. Tel.: (+49) 731 502 4385/4311, Fax: (+49) 731 502 4302. E-mail: thomas.gress@medizin.uni-ulm.de
HAHN, Stephan A.	Ruhr-Universitaet Bochum, Medizinische Klinik, Knappschaftskrankenhaus, Labor für Molekulare Onkologie In der Schornau 23-25, D-44892 Bochum, Germany. Tel.: (+49) 234/299-3464, Fax: (+49) 234/299-4380, E-mail: Stephan.A.Hahn@ruhr-uni-bochum.de
HOHEISEL, Joerg	Functional Genome Analysis, Deutsches Krebsforschungszentrum, Im Neuenheimer Feld 506, D-69120 Heidelberg, Germany Tel.: (+49) 6221 42-4680 Fax: (+49) 6221 42-4682 email: j.hoheisel@dkfz-heidelberg.de

LEMOINE, Nick — ICRF Molecular Oncology Unit, Dept of Cancer Medicine, Imperial College School of Medicine, Hammersmith Campus, Du Cane Road. London W12 0NN, UK.
Tel: (+44) 181 383 3975,
Fax: (+44) 181 383 3258
E-mail:N.Lemoine@icrf.icnet.uk

MALATS, Núria — Clinical & Molecular Epidemiology of Cancer Unit, Institut Municipal d'Investigacio Medica (IMIM), Universitat Pompeu Fabra
Carrer del Dr. Aiguader 80
E-08003 Barcelona, Spain
Tel.: (+34) 93 225 7553,
Fax: (+34) 93 221 3237

MOORE, Patrick — Dipartimento di Patologia - Anatomia Patologica, Università di Verona, Strada Le Grazie, I-37134 Verona, Italy
Tel. (+39) 045 8074 822,
Fax: (+39) 045 8098 136

MULERIS, Martine — UMR 147 CNRS, Institut Curie, 26 rue d'Ulm, F-75248 Paris Cedex 05, France
Tel: (+33) 1 42 34 66 75,
Fax: (+33) 1 42 34 66 74
E-mail: martine.muleris@curie.fr

PALOMERO, Teresa — Unitat de Biologia Cellular i Molecular, Institut Municipal d'Investigació Mèdica, Doctor Aiguader, 80, E-08003 Barcelona, Spain.
Tel.: (+34) 93 221 1009,
Fax: (+34) 93 221 3237

PARTSCH, Eva — Resource Center / Primary Database; German Human Genome Project at the Max Planck Institute for Molecular Genetics; Heubnerweg 6. D-14059 Berlin-Charlottenburg, Germany
Tel: (+49) 30 32639 100,
Fax: (+49) 30 32639 111
E-mail: partsch@rzpd.de

PAUL, Hubert — Abteilung Innere Medizin I, Universitätsklinikum Ulm, Robert Koch Str. 8, D-89081 Ulm, Germany
Tel.: (+49) 731 502 4311/4312,
Fax: (+49) 731 502 4302

PORTA, Miquel	Clinical & Molecular Epidemiology of Cancer Unit, Institut Municipal d'Investigacio Medica (IMIM), Universitat Autonoma de Barcelona Carrer del Dr. Aiguader 80 E-08003 Barcelona, Spain Tel.: (+34) 93 225 7553, Fax: (+34) 93 221 3237 E-mail: mporta@imim.es
RACZ, Gabor	Institute of Experimental Medicine, Hungarian Academy of Sciences, Szigony 43, H-1083 Budapest, Hungary. Tel: (+36) 1 210-0819/ ext. 133, Fax: (+36) 1 210-0813 E-mail: Racz@koli.hu
REAL, Francisco X.	Unitat de Biologia Cellular i Molecular, Institut Municipal d'Investigació Mèdica, Doctor Aiguader, 80, E-08003 Barcelona, Spain. Tel.: (+34) 93 221 1009, Fax: (+34) 93 221 3237 E-mail: preal@imim.es.
RIGAUD, Gildas	Dipartimento di Patologia - Anatomia Patologica, Università di Verona, Strada Le Grazie, I-37134 Verona, Italy. Tel.: (+39) 045 8074 822, Fax: (+39) 045 8098 136
SCARPA, Aldo	Dipartimento di Patologia - Anatomia Patologica, Università di Verona, Strada Le Grazie, I-37134 Verona, Italy. Tel.: (+39) 045 8074 822, Fax: (+39) 045 8098 136 E-mail: scarpa@anpat.univr.it
SCHWARZ, Sandra	Functional Genome Analysis, Deutsches Krebsforschungszentrum, Im Neuenheimer Feld 506, D-69120 Heidelberg, Germany. Tel: (+49) 622 142 4681, Fax: (+49) 622 142 4687 E-mail: sandra.schwarz@dkfz-heidelberg.de

SKOUDY, Anouchka — Unitat de Biologia Cellular i Molecular, Institut Municipal d'Investigació Mèdica, Doctor Aiguader, 80, E-08003 Barcelona, Spain.
Tel.: (+34) 93 221 1009,
Fax: (+34) 93 221 3237
E-mail: askoudy@imim.es

SOMMER, Gerrit — Abteilung Innere Medizin I, Universitätsklinikum Ulm, Robert Koch Str. 8, D-89081 Ulm, Germany
Tel.: (+49) 731 502 4311/4312,
Fax: (+49) 731 502 4302

TANIGUCHI, Tadaaki — ICRF Molecular Oncology Unit, Dept of Cancer Medicine, Imperial College School of Medicine, Hammersmith Campus, Du Cane Road. London W12 0NN, UK.
Tel: (+44) 181 383 3975,
Fax: (+44) 181 383 3258

VARGA, Gabor — Institute of Experimental Medicine, Hung. Acad. Sci., and Dept. Oral Biology, Semmelweis University of Medicine, Budapest, Hungary.
Tel: (+36) 1 210-0819/ ext 257 or 133,
Fax: (+36) 1 210-0813
E-mail: Varga-g@koki.hu

WENGER, Christoph — Abteilung Innere Medizin I, Universitätsklinikum Ulm, Robert Koch Str. 8, D-89081 Ulm, Germany
Tel.: (+49) 731 502 4311/4312,
Fax: (+49) 731 502 4302

Acknowledgements

The midterm meeting of the concerted action BMH4-CT98-3085, which is summarized in this proceedings book was a full success. I want to use this opportunity to acknowledge the effort of the group at the IMIM in Barcelona who organised this wonderful meeting. In particular I want to thank Francisco Real who volunteered to host this meeting in Barcelona, Leopoldo Español who took care to make it really happen, and Dr. J. Lloreta, L. Español and A.González for preparing the cover figure for this book.
At this point I want as well to thank our secretary, Erika Thanner, for the many hours she spent organising and administrating the project and for her help in editing this proceedings book.

T.M. Gress
Project Coordinator

Contents

Preface

T.M.Gress
Department of Internal Medicine I, Universitätsklinikum Ulm, 89081 Ulm, Germany

This book was written to summarize the midterm meeting of the concerted action BMH4-CT98-3085 funded by the European Union in the context of the BIOMEDII programme. The objective of this concerted action (CA) is to generate a European network allowing to share expertise, technologies and resources to speed up the process of characterisation of potential new disease genes in pancreatic cancer. The meeting in Barcelona in november 1999 was hosted by the group at the IMIM led by FX. Real, and was scheduled to allow a midterm evaluation of the indivdual projects. Around 30 scientists participated in this meeting, which took place in a relaxed atmosphere allowing a mutual exchange of data and experiences. This book includes a description of the concerted action, a state of the art article on the molecular biology of pancreatic cancer and brief articles summarizing the scientific presentations given by members of the individual groups. As the meeting provided a forum to present newest data and technologies, this book gives an excellent overview on some of the most actual developments in Europe concerning genetic alterations in pancreatic cancer.

The Editor

Molecular Pathogenesis of Pancreatic Cancer
T.M. Gress (Ed.)
IOS Press, 2000

The „concerted action"

T.M.Gress
Department of Internal Medicine I, Universitätsklinikum Ulm, 89081 Ulm, Germany

During the past few years members of the concerted action (CA) have used a variety of techniques to detect genetic alterations occuring at the levels of genomic DNA and of RNA in pancreatic cancer cells. The groups of T.Gress and H.Lehrach have employed a combination of array/chip-technology for expression profiling approaches to identify thousands of genes with pancreatic cancer specific gene expression [1]. The group of FX.Real used subtractive hybridisations to identify a number of genes overexpressed in pancreatic cancer cells but not in normal pancreatic epithelial cells [2]. Additional genes with pancreatic cancer-specific expression were isolated using representational difference analysis by the groups of T.Gress and JD.Hoheisel [3]. In addition several members of the CA have finalized projects aimed at identifying chromosomal alterations ocurring in pancreatic cancer. S.Hahn used allelotyping of pancreatic cancer nude mice xenografts to identify chromosomal areas of allelic loss [4]. This work finally led to the detection of a new tumour suppressor gene located at chromosome 18q21.1 denominated DPC4 (Deleted in Pancreatic Cancer) which is a part of the TGFβ signalling cascade [5]. Scarpa and collaborators used a combination of AP-PCR (arbitrarily-primed PCR) and microsatellite markers to identify a homozygous deletion and LOH (loss of heterozygosity) at chromosome 7q31.1-7q32 [6]. In a collaborative project with P.Lichter (DKFZ/Heidelberg) the group of T.Gress was involved in the mapping of chromosomal imbalances in pancreatic carcinoma by comparative genomic hybridisation [7]. This led to the identification of chromosomal areas with gains (potential amplifications) or loss (potential deletions) of chromosomal material. Among others the myb oncogene was identified as the relevant oncogene involved in an amplification on chromosome 6q24 [8].

Thus, during the years prior to the application of this concerted action members of the CA had identified a large number of genes with pancreatic cancer-specific expression and chromosomal areas amplified or deleted in pancreatic cancer. All genes involved in these alterations represent potential disease-associated genes or disease genes as e.g. oncogenes or tumour suppressor genes. It will be the main task of the next years to device procedures allowing to use this selection of candidate disease genes to identify respectively select genes associated with processes relevant for cancerogenesis in the pancreas as e.g. tumour cell proliferation, differentiation, metastasis and invasion. In addition, specific strategies and technologies will have to be developed and applied allowing a structural and functional characterisation of these genes. These research tasks comprise a considerable amount of work and the application, respectively development of complex technologies. No single laboratory will be able to provide the resources, facilities, technologies and the man power required for these research tasks. Thus, a close collaboration of European groups working in the same field including the joint use of resources, facilities and scientifc expertise is mandatory.

To accomplish these goals we created a network of basic molecular/cytogenetic and oncological research groups, interested in the identification and characterisation of potential disease genes. By making specialized techniques, resources and facilities accessible to all members of the CA and by allowing personnel exchange for targeted training we expect, that this network will contribute to accelerate the understanding of tumourigenesis in the pancreas and to identify new disease genes.

Literature

[1] T.M. Gress et al, A pancreatic cancer-specific expression profile. Oncogene **13** (1996) 1819-1830.

[2] R.Paciucci *et al*, Isolation of tissue-type plasminogen activator, cathepsin H, and non-specific cross-reacting antigen from SK-PC-1 pancreas cancer cells using subtractive hybridisation. FEBS-Lett. **385** (1996) 72-6.

[3] T.M. Gress *et al*, Identification of genes with pancreatic cancer-specific expression by use of cDNA representational difference analysis. Genes.Chrom.Cancer **19** (1997) 97-103.

[4] A.Achille *et al*, Chromosome 7q allelic losses in pancreatic carcinoma. Cancer Res. **56** (1996).

[5] S. Hahn *et al*, Allelotype of pancreatic adenocarcinoma using xenograft enrichment. Cancer Res. **55** (1995) 4670-46775.

[6] S. Solinas-Toldo *et al*, Mapping of chromosomal imbalances in pancreatic carcinoma by comparative genomic hybridisation. Cancer Res.**56** (1996) 3803-3807.

[7] C.Wallrapp *et al*, Characterization of a high copy number amplification at 6q24 in pancreatic cancer identifies myb as candidate oncogene. Cancer Res. **57** (1997) 3135-3139.

[8] T.M. Gress *et al*, European Pancreatic Cancer Reference Library System (EPCRLS). Europ.J.Cancer, **30A** (1994) 1391-1394.

Molecular Pathogenesis of Pancreatic Cancer
T.M. Gress (Ed.)
IOS Press, 2000

Molecular profile of pancreatic cancer

Nicholas R. Lemoine, Vorapan Sirivatanauksorn, Tatjana Crnogorac-Jurcevic
ICRF Molecular Oncology Unit, Dept of Cancer Medicine, Imperial College School of Medicine, Hammersmith Campus, Du Cane Road. London W12 0NN, UK

As a result of the application of modern molecular biological techniques to cell systems *in vitro* and human tumours *in vivo*, there is increasing information about the genetic basis of cancer. The development and growth of pancreatic adenocarcinoma involves oncogene activation, loss of tumour suppressor gene function, and overexpression of receptor-ligand systems (Figure 1).

Oncogenes and Growth Factor Systems Implicated

KRAS

KRAS is one of the three members of the human RAS gene family that code for highly related 21-kDa proteins with guanosine triphosphatase (GTPase) activity. It was first identified as the transforming principle of the Kirsten strains of rat sarcoma virus and has been assigned to the short arm of chromosome 12 (12p12.1-pter). RAS proteins which are synthesised in the cytosol and attached to the inner side of the plasma membrane after posttranslational modifications, have functional and structural resemblance to the regulatory (G) proteins. It has now been shown that they play a role in transduction of signals from the cell surface.

Naturally occurring mutations in KRAS oncogene have been localised to codons 12, 13, and 61. The presence of a glycine residue at codon 12 appears to be necessary for the normal function of RAS proteins. Substitution of glycine by any other amino acid residue (with the exception of proline) results in the oncogenic activation of these molecules. The mutants result in a reduced rate of guanosine triphosphate (GTP) hydrolysis and a resistance to the inhibitory effects of GTPase-activating proteins (GAPs). The mutant RAS proteins are therefore locked into an active GTP-bound state and transmit a constitutive growth signal to the nucleus. The incidence of mutated KRAS genes varies widely among different tumour types. The highest incidence is found in pancreatic carcinomas and since 1988 more than 50 reports have described KRAS mutation in this tumour type. RAS mutations are also found frequently in colorectal carcinomas, adenocarcinomas of lung and follicular and undifferentiated thyroid carcinomas, whereas in several other tumour types a mutated gene is only occasionally found [1]. The KRAS mutations present in pancreatic carcinomas are almost exclusively at codon 12 and analysis of the specific nucleotide reveals a heterogeneous type of mutation [2]. This might be caused by multiple carcinogens and/or diverse errors during DNA replication and repair rather than a single, specific mutagen. The most common mutation at codon 12 is a transition second base from guanine to adenine (GGT---GAT), similar to those in colorectal tumours, while guanine to thymine (G to T) transversion (GGT---GTT) is more prevalent in lung carcinomas. In contrast, the aspartic acid mutation at codon 13 (GGC----GAC) is relatively frequent in colorectal tumours but rare in pancreatic and lung carcinomas [2].

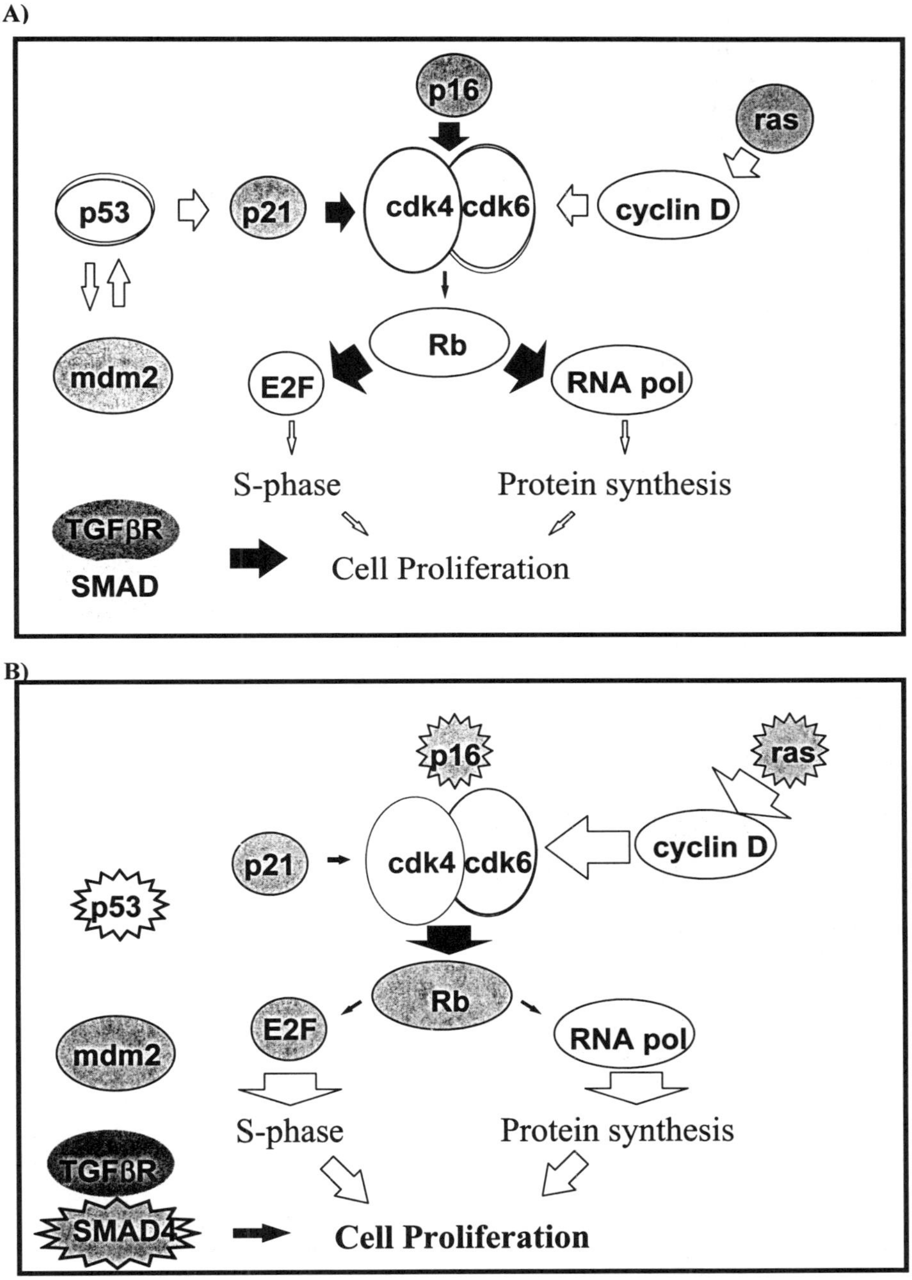

Figure 1. Cell-cycle regulatory pathway in normal cells (A) and in the development of pancreatic cancer cells (B). Disruption of p53 or p16 and mutation of the KRAS oncogene abrogates the control of the cyclin-dependent kinases (cdk) and retinoblastoma (Rb) gene pathway, causing continuous growth of the pancreatic tumour.
(⇨ upregulation; ➡ downregulation)

The differences in the mutation spectrum of the KRAS gene in cancers of the gastrointestinal and respiratory tracts are suggestive of differential exposure to genotoxic agents. The mutation in pancreatic cancer may be produced by a different type of carcinogen, such as aromatic amines and *N*-nitrosamines while benzpyrene, a tobacco carcinogen, is thought to be the cause in lung cancers [3]. Moreover, a recent study showed the prevalence of KRAS mutation in cases associated with alcohol consumption (one of the risk factors for pancreatic carcinoma) was 3 times higher than in non-drinkers [4]. In addition, the mutational pattern in cancers of the different European countries, and also when compared with Japanese, shows remarkable differences, both in the site of the mutation (first or second base) and in the ratio of transitions over transversions.

KRAS mutations are also found in other pancreatic tumours of ductal origin such as cystadenoma, cystadenocarcinoma [5], and intraductal papillary mucinous tumours (IPMT) [6]. Recently, one study showed a stepwise increase in the frequency of KRAS mutations at codon 12 correlated with the stage of neoplastic evolution to cancer [7]. The mutations are observed as frequently in patients with IPMT (81%) as in patients with pancreatic carcinomas. They found a relatively high number of guanine to cytosine (G to C) transversion in IPMT, different from the guanine to adenine (G to A), the commonest base change in pancreatic cancer.

Since the majority of pancreatic carcinomas have mutated KRAS gene, the presence of the mutation has been proposed as a molecular genetic marker for malignancy. Several studies [8,9] reported that detection of KRAS mutations in fine needle aspirates of pancreatic lesions increases the sensitivity of the diagnosis for this cancer. The detection of KRAS mutation in pancreatic juice, bile, peripheral blood and also in stool samples has been reported [10,11]. However, KRAS mutations are not only found in pancreatic carcinomas but also in mucinous hypertrophy and ductal papillary hyperplasia [12,11]. A recent study also found a high frequency of KRAS mutations in hyperplastic ducts associated with chronic pancreatitis [13]. This provides a genetic basis for the potential progression of chronic pancreatitis to pancreatic carcinoma and suggests that KRAS mutations are an early event in pancreatic carcinogenesis. Although the risk of pancreatic cancer was significantly increased in patients with chronic pancreatitis with the cumulative risk of 1.8% and 4% at 10 and 20 years after diagnosis of pancreatitis [14], a recent study reported that the finding of KRAS mutation in patients with chronic pancreatitis had no direct clinical relevance to the development of pancreatic cancer during a follow up of 140 months [15].

It appears that in the absence of a cooperating genetic event, such as inactivation of the tumour suppressor gene p16, the lesions containing cells with KRAS mutations are self-limiting (by apoptosis after a strictly limited member of cell divisions, as shown by transfection experiments [16] and the risk of progression to full malignancy is probably around 1% or less. Likewise, a recent study suggested that inactivating mutations of the p16 gene following the KRAS mutation may contribute to the progression of pancreatic carcinoma [17]. The presence of KRAS mutations does not appear to be a useful prognostic marker in pancreatic carcinoma. While the survival rate of lung cancers was positively correlated with the absence of KRAS mutations [18], and G to T and G to C transversions conferred poor prognosis than G to A transitions in colonic carcinomas [19], no correlations were found between KRAS genotype and tumour size, histological grade, tumour ploidy, tumour proliferation index, or patient survival in pancreatic carcinomas [20].

Epidermal growth factor receptor family

Epidermal growth factor (EGF) receptor (EGFR) (also known as c-erbB) is a transmembrane protein with intrinsic tyrosine kinase activity which is involved in normal cellular growth and differentiation. The EGFR gene is usually overexpressed at high levels in pancreatic adenocarcinoma due to increased gene transcription [21]. To date, at least 15 EGF-like ligands have been described including transforming growth factor alpha (TGFα), amphiregulin (AR), heparin-binding EGF-like growth factor (HB-EGF), betacellulin, and epiregulin. These ligands form a complex series of interactions with different members of the EGF receptor family that promote either homo- or hetero-dimerisation [22]. EGF is a potent mitogenic stimulus for cells in different tissues including pancreatic cells [23]. A recent report shows that EGF evoked a strong proliferative response in all cell types studied in the pancreas [24]. Pancreatic carcinomas overexpress EGF and TGFα (12-46% and 50-95% of cases respectively) compared to normal human pancreas tissue [25,26]. It was shown that human pancreatic cancers exhibit increased EGF and TGFα immunostaining [26]. Furthermore, coexpression of the receptor and both EGF and TGFα ligands is found in 20% of pancreatic tumours, and coexpression of the receptor and one of the two ligands in 18% more [27]. In the normal pancreas, AR appears to be in the nuclei of ductal cells, while it is also present in the cytoplasm of the ductal adenocarcinoma cells [28]. There is a significant correlation among cytoplasmic AR immunoreactivity in pancreatic cancer tissues, advanced tumour stage and shorter post-operative survival [29]. In a recent study, AR has been shown to have the potential to act as an autocrine growth factor in pancreatic cancer cells [30]. *In vitro*, HB-EGF enhanced the growth of human pancreatic cancer cell lines in a dose-dependent manner, with a potency that was generally similar to that of EGF and TGFα. Immunohistochemical analysis revealed the presence of HB-EGF immunoreactivity in pancreatic cancer cells in 50% of the tumours [31]. Epiregulin is a novel EGF family member which exhibits bifunctional regulatory properties as it stimulates the growth of many types of cells including fibroblasts and hepatocytes, while inhibiting the growth of several epithelial tumour cells [32]. The concomitant overexpression of the EGFR and one or more of its ligands appears to be a marker of poor prognosis and has been correlated with enhanced ability of certain tumour to invade normal tissue, to metastasise, and a shorter postoperative survival period [27].

EGFR belongs to a family of closely related transmembrane proteins that include HER-2/neu (also known as c-erbB-2), HER3 (c-erbB-3), and HER4 (c-erbB-4). HER-2/neu appears to be required to act in heterodimers with other family member, whereas HER3 and HER4 bind to the family of heregulins. In additions, HER4 also binds to betacellulin, a potent mitogen produced by the β cells of the islets of Langerhans. It has been shown that HER-2/neu, and HER3 are frequently overexpressed in pancreatic cancers [33,34]. There are various data concerning the incidence of HER-2/neu expression in invasive ductal adenocarcinomas [33,25] and in intraductal mucin-hypersecreting neoplasms of the pancreas [35]. A recent study showed that the pattern of HER-2/neu expression was related to glandular differentiation and early oncogenesis of pancreatic cancer, but not related to survival differences [36]. In contrast, HER3 was found to be associated with advanced tumour stage and shorter postoperative survival [37].

Hepatocyte growth factor and MET receptor

Hepatocyte growth factor (HGF), otherwise known as scatter factor (SF), is a ligand for the c-met protooncogene product of receptor tyrosine kinase. It is a mesenchymal- or stromal-derived multipotent polypeptide which mediates epithelial-mesenchymal interactions. HGF has been implicated in the regulation of mitogenesis, motogenesis, and morphogenesis. *In vivo*, it plays a role in tissue regeneration, tumour progression, and embryological processes, which generally require both cell motility and cell proliferation. Over the past few years, the structure, function and signal transduction pathways of HGF and its receptor have become clearer. It is now known to take important parts in the regulation of both normal physiological processes as well as pathological ones [38].

HGF is detectable at low levels in the normal human exocrine pancreas, but it is up-regulated ten-fold in the majority of pancreatic ductal adenocarcinoma [39]. The MET receptor has also been observed to have weak expression in normal pancreas but markedly increased in pancreatic carcinoma [40]. This supports the assumption that HGF could act as a growth promoting factor for this cancer. *In vitro*, phosphorylation of the MET receptor in human pancreas cell lines caused by HGF stimulates their movements. If there is overexpression of MET receptor, constitutive autophosphorylation can occur even in the absence of exogenous ligand. It can be concluded that upregulation of this system may stimulate growth and enhance motility and therefore be an important step in the progression of metastatic spread [39,40,41].

Transforming growth factor beta family

The transforming growth factor beta (TGFβ) superfamily consists of large numbers of regulatory polypeptides which include several TGFβ isoforms as well as activin, inhibin, bone morphogenetic proteins (BMPs), Mullerian inhibiting substance (MIS), and growth and differentiation factors (GDFs). Three isoforms of TGFβ (TGFβ1, TGFβ2, and TGFβ3) exist in mammals. TGFβs possess three major activities: they inhibit proliferation of most cells, but can stimulate the growth of some mesenchymal cells; they exert immunosuppressive effects; and they enhance extracellular matrix formation. All three TGFβ isoforms are expressed in both the exocrine and endocrine constituents of normal pancreas. TGFβ1 protein expression was present in a large number of acinar cells, whereas TGFβ2 and TGFβ3 immunoreactivity was more intense in islets, and all three isoforms have the same intensity of immunostaining in ductal cells [42]. In human pancreatic cancers, there are increased levels of TGFβ isoforms and enhanced TGFβ mRNA expression [43]. Only the expression of the TGFβ2 isoform correlated with advanced tumour stage indicating that in pancreatic cancer the presence of the TGFβ2 isoform may be a marker for progression [42]. Nevertheless, increased TGFβ expression may also occur in degenerating nonneoplastic cells next to the invasive tumour. This suggests that the upregulation of the TGFβ isoforms should not be considered to be tumour-specific [44].

There are three major receptors: TGFβRI, TGFβRII, and TGFβRIII. Two types of the receptors (type I and type II) possessing a serine/threonine kinase activity within their cytoplasmic domains are involved in signal transduction. Overexpression of TGFβRII may result from both increased gene transcription rate or prolonged TGFβRII mRNA stability in pancreatic cancer cells *in vivo*, whereas TGFβRIII mRNA levels are not increased. Thus, enhanced levels of TGFβRII may have a role in regulating human pancreatic cancer cell growth, while TGFβRIII may function in the extracellular matrix [44].

Fibroblast growth factors and receptors

The fibroblast growth factors (FGF) are a family of structurally related polypeptides that are mitogenic for a broad range of cell type as well as mediators of a wide spectrum of developmental and pathophysiological processes *in vivo* and *in vitro*.

The FGF family presently comprises eighteen members (FGF1-18). FGF1 (acidic) and FGF2 (basic) are closely related prototypes of this family; each is chemotactic toward fibroblasts, participates in tissue repair, and promotes angiogenesis. They are detected at low levels in the normal pancreas and exhibit increased expression at the mRNA levels in chronic pancreatitis [45]. There is increased expression of FGF1 and FGF2 in pancreatic carcinomas (60% and 50% of cases respectively). These appear to be a significant correlation between the expression of either FGF1 or FGF2 in the cancer cells and advanced tumour stage [46].

FGFs stimulate cellular response by binding to and activating a family of transmembrane receptors tyrosine kinases. There are four distinct high-affinity FGF receptors (FGFR1-4). FGFR1 and FGFR2 are expressed in a wide variety of cell types while FGFR3 and FGFR4 have a more restricted pattern of expression. In the normal pancreas, all FGFRs are found at relatively low levels, whereas significant expression of FGFR1, 3 and 4 is found in approximately 60% of pancreatic cancers [47]. A recent study also found that the expression of FGF2 in human pancreatic carcinoma is strongly associated with the proliferation of tumour cells and intratumour endothelial cells and its increased expression may give tumour cells a growth advantage [48].

Vascular endothelial growth factor

Vascular endothelial growth factor (VEGF), also known as vascular permeability factor (VPF), is an endothelial cell-specific mitogen and a regulator of physiological and pathological angiogenesis. The VEGF family comprises secreted homodimeric proteins encoded by a single gene. Alternative splicing of VEGF pre-mRNA leads to four isoforms having 121,165, 189 and 206 amino acids residue in the mature monomer. All four forms are mitogenic to vascular endothelial cells and induce vascular permeabilisation. VEGF signals through two high-affinity transmembrane receptors which are class III transmembrane protein tyrosine kinases. VEGF receptor-1 was originally named the fms-like tyrosine kinase, and is also known as flt-1. VEGF receptor-2, also known as KDR, is the human homologue of flk-1.

VEGF expression has been demonstrated in a number of human cancer cell lines suggesting a trophic role for VEGF in supporting tumour growth *via* host angiogenesis. In normal pancreatic tissue, VEGF immunoreactivity was found in islet cells which are known to express and secrete VEGF [49]. In duct ligation-induced acute pancreatitis, numerous inflammatory leucocytes containing VEGF were seen to infiltrate between hyperplastic ducts [50]. This indicates the possibility that VEGF plays a role in the paracrine regulation of ductal growth and differentiation. A recent study showed 5.2-fold increase in VEGF mRNA transcript in pancreatic cancer samples in comparison with normal pancreatic tissues. This finding was associated with increased blood vessel number, larger tumour size, and enhanced local spread but not with decreased patient survival [51]. Hence this factor may contribute to the angiogenic process and tumour growth in this disease.

Retinoids and receptors

Retinoids are natural and synthetic derivatives of vitamin A. They elicit a large array of biological responses during morphogenesis and differentiation. Similar to the steroid hormone superfamily, the pleiotrophic biological effects of retinoids are mediated by two families of nuclear retinoic acid (RA) receptor, the RA receptors and the retinoid x receptors, each consisting of three receptors subtypes of α, β, and γ. Both receptors act as ligand-activated transcription factors, controlling gene transcription initiated from promotors of retinoid-regulated genes by interacting with cis-acting DNA elements, the so called RA responsive elements [52].

There has been increasing evidence that the RA and vitamin D are naturally occurring agents controlling cellular differentiation and proliferation both in normal and malignant cells. *In vitro*, it has been shown that vitamin D analogues together with retinoids inhibit the growth of human pancreatic cancer cells [53]. In addition, a recent study found that retinoids decrease pancreatic carcinoma cell adhesion to laminin, one of the major constituents of basement membranes, which results in growth inhibition [54]. RA receptor β expression (RARβ) is known to be lost or decreased during malignant transformation in human pancreatic adenocarcinoma [55]. One study suggested that overexpression of RARβ in human pancreatic carcinoma cells inhibited cellular proliferation *in vitro* and *in vivo* [56]. Exploitation of RAR expression may provide rational strategies for retinoid treatment of pancreatic cancer in the future.

AKT2

AKT2 was identified as one of the human homologues of the *v-akt* oncogene. Human AKT2 is located at 19q13.1-q13.2 and encodes a protein-serine/threonine kinase which has significant sequence and structural homology to members of the protein kinase C and cyclic adenosine monophophate-dependent protein kinase families. It is activated by platelet-derived growth factor, EGF, FGF2, and insulin through phosphatidylinositol-3-OH kinase, suggesting that it is an important signal mediator that may contribute to the control of cell proliferation and malignant transformation. It has been shown to be amplified or overexpressed in approximately 10% of primary tumours and cell lines of pancreatic cancer [57]. Interestingly, this study also showed the reduction of tumour growth and invasiveness in pancreatic tumour cell lines transfected with antisense AKT2 RNA. Such results suggests that antisense inhibition of AKT2 may be a potentially important approach for pancreatic cancer gene therapy.

Tumour Suppressor Genes

P53

The p53 gene is located on the short arm of chromosome 17 (17p13) and encodes a 53 kDa nuclear phosphoprotein (p53 protein) which functions as a transcription factor. In response to DNA damage, p53 appears to direct the transcription of the p21 WAF1 gene, which is an inhibitor of cyclin-dependent kinases. This suggests that p53-dependent p21 induction is responsible for arresting the cell cycle in G1 following DNA damage. Moreover, p53 protein is also required to direct cells into apoptosis when the level of DNA damage is too great.

Inactivation of the p53 gene is the most common genetic alteration found in human malignancies, and mutations and/or deletions occur very frequently in pancreatic carcinomas (40-70% of cases) [58,59]. Transitions represent the majority of the point mutations (70%) in pancreatic cancers, while transversions (which have been seen at high frequency in smoking-related carcinomas such as lung, oesophageal, and head and neck tumours) were not common. Most mutations in pancreatic carcinomas affect G:C sites with a predominance of transitions (70%), mainly represented by G:C to A:T substitutions, which is reminiscent of the pattern observed in colonic carcinomas (75% of transitions) [59]. Unlike other cancers such as liver and colonic cancers, no specific site seems to be preferentially affected in p53 mutations of pancreatic cancers. The missense mutations are scattered through numerous codons, such as at 135, 158-160, 248, 273, 282 and 286, but are mainly confined to four regions of the gene that are conserved through evolution, located in exons 5-8. There is a peculiar preference for pancreatic carcinomas to have intragenic deletions, and in particular 1-2 base-pair microdeletions. These deletions frequently were within repeated runs of single nucleotides or nucleotide pairs.

Due to an increased half life and accumulation of p53 protein caused by p53 mutation, p53 protein concentrations in serum of pancreatic cancer patients are significantly higher than in chronic pancreatitis patients or healthy persons. The concentrations are also reported to be significantly higher in tumours with distant metastases than without metastases [60], results similar to findings in colonic and lung cancers [61,62]. Thus, serum p53 protein concentrations may be an additional tumour marker in pancreatic cancer patients.

p16 (MTS1/CDKN2/CDKN41/p16^{INK4a}/DPC3)

p16 is one of the inhibitors for cyclin-dependent kinases (CDKs) which complexes with cyclin D1 and drive a cell's progression through the division cycle. p16 acts on RB1 to form a negative feedback loop that regulates the ability of RB1 to prevent cell proliferation. Deletions or mutations in the p16 gene may affect the relative balance of functional p16 and cyclin D, resulting in abnormal cell growth. It consists of three exons which encode a 148 amino acid-protein of MW 16 kDa. Mutations of the p16 gene occur in pancreatic cancer at a rate of 30-82%, higher than that reported in any other tumour type [63]. Although the RB1, p16, cyclin D1 and CDK4 pathway in other tumour types can be abrogated by inactivation of any of members of the pathway, in pancreatic carcinoma this pathway appears to be almost exclusively inactivated by alterations of the p16 protein [64]. Thus, p16 inactivations involve a strong tissue-specificity. p16 is located at chromosome 9p21, a region that is linked to familial melanoma and homozygously deleted in many tumour cell lines [65,66]. Of interest, this gene may play a major role as a tumour suppressor gene in a subset of the familial atypical mole-multiple melanoma (FAMMM) syndrome with pancreatic cancer.

A portion of the INK4a gene was found to have the capacity to encode a second growth-inhibitory protein, p19^{ARF} (ARF stands for alternative-reading-frame protein) [67]. This unique gene structure generates two distinct open reading frames (ORFs) that initiate in different first exons and continue in alternative reading frames in a common second exon. The overlapping exonic sequences enables this gene to encode two completely unrelated protein products. Thus, the INK4a gene is therefore defined as the INK4a/ARF locus. ARF stabilises p53 by promoting the degradation of MDM2 proto-oncogene. Thus, point mutations and biallelic deletions are functionally distinct and may have been selectively targeted during tumour development, since the INK4a mutations selectively inactive the Rb pathway and the deletion of the ARF-INK4a locus impairs both Rb and p53 pathways [68].

The p16 alterations in pancreatic carcinomas may be caused by a number of mechanisms, including hetero- or homo-zygous deletions, coding sequence mutations, and transcriptional silencing. Loss of function usually occur by loss of heterozygosity (90%) or homozygous deletion (40%) which frequently extends to involve another candidate suppressor gene p15 (MTS2) at a closely adjacent locus. Homozygous co-deletion of p16 and p15 has been reported at the rate of 46% in pancreatic cancers [69]. p15 also acts as an effector of TGFβ-induced cell-cycle arrest and may be important in pancreatic carcinogenesis, though there is no direct evidence of p15 being a tumour suppressor gene.

Gene deleted in pancreatic carcinoma, locus 4 (DPC4) (SMAD4)

In one study, 48% of pancreatic carcinomas were found to have homozygous deletions at the site 18q21.1 [70]. Because this was the fourth locus to be investigated for this special form of deletion in pancreatic cancer, the cloned gene was initially named

DPC4. The coding sequence of this gene is 1660 nucleotides in length, covering 11 exons. It is very similar (75% to 85% at the sequence level) to a Drosophila gene, *mothers against dpp* (MAD) which is needed in early fly development, and so DPC4 has now been renamed SMAD4. It cascades a component of the signal transduction pathway for the TGFβ superfamily of receptors, which usually act to promote differentiation and to slow the growth of cells. A recent study in breast cancer cells showed that SMAD4 is involved in growth inhibition and plasminogen activator inhibitor 1 (PAI-1) induction [71]. Moreover, it has been shown that this gene contains a transcriptional activation domain [72]. Mutations at this gene are frequently detected in sporadic pancreatic cancer, including nonsense mutation in exons 8, 9, 11, missense mutation at exon 11, and splice donor site mutation after exon 10 [73]. However, no DPC4 mutations were found in the germline DNA of 25 individuals (8 with pancreatic carcinoma) from 11 kindreds with a familial history of pancreatic carcinoma. Thus, DPC4 does not appear to be a candidate for the gene responsible for the familial form of pancreatic carcinoma [74]. DPC4 is also believed to be an important target gene promoting tumourigenesis of non-functional neuroendocrine pancreatic carcinomas, and extremely rare type of pancreatic cancer, as 55% of the cases revealed mutations of this gene [75].

Other tumour suppressor genes

The Retinoblastoma (Rb) gene is located at 13q14 and is an important tumour suppressor gene found to be mutated in numerous tumour types. However, inactivation of Rb rarely occurs in pancreatic carcinoma. A study showed evidence of Rb allele loss in only two of 32 (6%) pancreatic cancers and no evidence for loss of the gene deleted in colorectal carcinoma (DCC) was found [76]. Thus, the alterations of Rb and DCC are unlikely to play a major role in pancreatic carcinogenesis. There have been reports of a high prevalence of allelic imbalance and loci noted to be homozygously deleted in pancreatic cancer, which have been labeled DPC loci 1 and 2. These colocalise at the 13q12 region of the breast cancer gene, BRCA2. Suspicions are therefore raised that the BRCA2 gene might represent the pancreatic cancer tumour suppressor gene on 13q and there is evidence that breast cancers and pancreatic cancers can have a shared pattern of inheritance. The germline BRCA2 mutations were reported in 7.3% of patients with apparently sporadic adenocarcinoma of the pancreas [77]. Recently, the STK11/LKB1 Peutz-Jeghers tumour suppressor gene which is on distal chromosome 19p was biallelic inactivated in a pancreatic cancer of a patient with the Peutz-Jeghers syndrome and in 4-6% of sporadic pancreatic and biliary adenocarcinomas. The germline and somatic genetic alterations of the STK11/LKB1 gene may play a role in carcinogenesis of pancreatic cancer [78].

Telomerase

Telomerase is an enzyme that contains an RNA template complementary to GGTTAG repeats and is believed to be involved in the *de novo* synthesis of GGTTAG telomeric DNA onto chromosomal ends. Almost all normal somatic cells have no detectable telomerase activity except for proliferative cells of self-renewal tissues such as haematopoietic progenitor cells, lymphocytes, skin basal cells, and intestinal stem cells. Activation and stabilisation of telomerase are considered to be necessary for immortalisation of human tumour cells. Telomerase activity is (at higher frequency) detected in a wide range of cancers such as neuroblastomas (94%), lung cancers (80%), colorectal cancers (93%), hepatocellular carcinoma (85%), gastric cancers (85%), and breast cancers (93%). In pancreatic carcinoma, it was detected in 95-100% of cases but was detectable in none of the benign pancreatic tumours examined [79]. This suggests that telomerase activity may play a role in pancreatic carcinogenesis. Moreover, eight *ex vivo* brushing samples of the duct of pancreatic cancers demonstrated telomerase activity, whereas no detectable activity in four samples of benign lesions [79]. Thus, telomerase activity may be a specific marker and detection in brushing samples or pancreatic juice may be useful in the early diagnosis of this tumour.

Modern approach to explore novel genetic events in pancreatic cancer

The genetic study of pancreatic adenocarcinoma has been greatly hindered by the technical difficulties presented by the characteristic host desmoplastic reaction to the tumours. Contaminating non-neoplastic cells often preclude the detection of the genetic events involved in tumourigenesis. To enrich for the neoplastic cell population, an indirect method to analyse pancreatic adenocarcinoma through the use of xenografted tumours was developed [80]. At the time of surgery, 1-2 mm pieces of primary tissue are implanted into severe combined immunodeficient (SCID) mice. The xenografts are harvested at a tumour size of 1.0 cm in diameter. Histological comparison of primary and xenograft tumours revealed that the degree of differentiation and nuclear pleomorphism was, in general, retained. Consistent results were shown when the integrity of the xenograft explants were analysed by comparison of allele loss analyses and p16/INK4a mutation analysis. Eighteen xenografted tumours of pancreatic adenocarcinoma were used in a PCR-based allelotype using 283 polymorphic markers and an average coverage of 4.1 informative markers per chromosomal arm per case. Highly frequent allelic loss (more than 60%) was detected at chromosomes 1p, 9p, 17p, and 18q. Moderately frequent allelic loss (40-60%) was detected at 3p, 6p, 6q, 8p, 10q, 12q, 13q, 18p, 21q, and 22q [80].

Sample preparation is one of the most important step for the molecular biological analysis. The presence of surrounding or infiltrating normal cells, especially in pancreatic cancer, can negatively impact on the results. Many techniques including needle-based microdissection and irradiating the unwanted surrounding cells in a tissue slide have been successfully used to isolate a few hundred cells from heterogeneous tissue samples. However, they are time-consuming, labour-intensive and require a high degree of manual skill. A laser capture microdissection (LCM) system, a novel membrane-based microdissection technique, has been developed by Liotta's group [81]. The method entails placing a sterile transparent film over a tissue section, visualising the tissue microscopically, and selectively adhering the cells of interest to the film with a fixed-position, short-duration, focused pulse from an infrared laser. Because more than 90% of the laser radiation is absorbed within the thermoplastic film, little direct heating of the tissue specimen occurred. The film with the procured tissue is then removed from the section and placed directly into DNA, RNA, or enzyme buffer for processing. Because laser beams can be focused to a one-cell diameter (about 10 μm), transfer of a targeted single cell among the hundreds of different cell types in a tumour specimen appears possible with this technique.

Previously, the identification of mutant genes relied on positional cloning. A number of "genome scanning" techniques have been reported which are predominantly based around the polymerase chain reaction (PCR) and used by several laboratories in order to identify candidate genes involved in cancer. Representational Difference Analysis (RDA) is a method for finding the differences between complex genomes (*eg* tumour and normal) [82]. One of the numerous applications of RDA is the cloning of probes for the detection of genetic lesions in cancer. RDA raises the efficiency of subtractive hybridisation by combining it with two additional elements: representation and kinetic enrichment. Representations are generated by a PCR-based size selection applied to the restriction fragments of both genomes. The tester DNA sample is prepared from normal DNA and the driver DNA sample from pure tumour DNA derived from the same patient. In this way, RDA generates probes that can detect different types of DNA alterations in tumours. Using this approach, the DPC4/SMAD4 tumour suppressor gene has been identified [73]. Another fragment isolated with the RDA approach (DPC1) led to the identification of the breast cancer susceptibility locus, BRCA2 [83].

References

[1] Bos JL. ras oncogenes in human cancer: a review. *Cancer Res.* **49**, (1989) 4682-4689.

[2] Capella G, *et al.* Frequency and spectrum of mutations at codons 12 and 13 of the c-K-ras gene in human tumors. *Environ. Health Perspect.* **93**, (1991) 125-131.

[3] Fujii H, *et al.* Pancreatic ductal adenocarcinomas induced in Syriam hamsters by N-nitrosobis(2-oxopropyl) amine contain a c-Ki-ras oncogene with a point-mutated codon 12. *Mol. Carcinog.* **3**, (1990) 296-301.

[4] Malats N, *et al.* Ki-ras mutations in exocrine pancreatic cancer: association with clinico-pathological characteristics and with tobacco and alcohol consumption. *Int. J. Cancer* **70**, (1997) 661-667.

[5] Yanagisawa A, *et al.* c-Ki-ras point mutations in ductectatic-type mucinous cystic neoplasms of the pancreas. *Jpn. J. Cancer Res.* **82**, (1991) 1057-1060.

[6] Hoshi T, Imai M, Ogawa K,. Frequent K-ras mutations and absence of p53 mutations in mucin-producing tumors of the pancreas. *J Surg Oncol* **55**, (1994) 84-91.

[7] Z'graggen K, *et al.* Prevalence of activating K-ras mutations in the evolutionary stages of neoplasia in intraductal papillary mucinous tumors of the pancreas. *Ann. Surg.* **226**, (1997) 491-500.

[8] Evans, DB *et al.* Molecular diagnosis of exocrine pancreatic cancer using a percutaneous technique. *Ann. Surg. Oncol.* **3**, (1996) 241-246.

[9] Villanueva A. *et al.* Diagnostic utility of K-ras mutations in fine-needle aspirates of pancreatic masses. *Gastroenterology* **110**, (1996) 1587-1594.

[10] Tada M, *et al.* Detection of ras gene mutations in pancreatic juice and peripheral blood of patients with pancreatic adenocarcinoma. *Cancer Res.* **53**, (1993) 2472-2474.

[11] Caldas C, *et al.* Detection of K-ras mutations in the stool of patients with pancreatic adenocarcinoma and pancreatic ductal hyperplasia. *Cancer Res.* **54**, (1994) 3568-3573.

[12] DiGiuseppe JA, *et al.* (1994) Detection of K-ras mutations in mucinous pancreatic duct hyperplasia from a patient with a family history of pancreatic carcinoma. *Am. J. Pathol.* **144,** (1994) 889-895.

[13] Rivera JA, *et al.* Analysis of K-ras oncogene mutations in chronic pancreatitis with ductal hyperplasia. *Surgery* **121**, (1997) 42-49.

[14] Lowenfels AB, *et al.* Pancreatitis and the risk of pancreatic cancer. International pancreatitis study group. *N. Engl. J. Med.* **328**, (1993) 1433-1437.

[15] Furuya N, *et al.* Long-term follow-up of patients with chronic pancreatitis and K-ras gene mutation detected in pancreatic juice. *Gastroenterology* **113**, (1997) 593-598.

[16] Burns J, *et al. In vitro* transformation of epithelial cells by ras oncogenes. *Epithelial Cell Biol.* **2**, (1993) 26-43.

[17] Moskaluk CA, Hruban RH, Kern SE,. p16 and K-ras gene mutations in the intraductal precursors of human pancreatic adenocarcinoma. *Cancer Res.* **57**, (1997a) 2140-2143.

[18] Silini EM, *et al.* K-ras gene mutations: an unfavorable prognostic marker in stage I lung adenocarcinoma. *Virchows Arch.* **424**, (1994) 367-373.

[19] Moerkerk P, *et al.* Type and number of Ki-ras point mutations relate to stage of human colorectal cancer. *Cancer Res.* **54,** (1994) 3376-3378.

[20] Motojima K, *et al.* Mutations in the Kirsten-ras oncogene are common but lack correlation with prognosis and tumor stage in human pancreatic carcinoma. *Am. J. Gastroenterol.* **86**, (1991) 1784-1788.

[21] Lemoine NR, *et al.* The epidermal growth factor receptor in human pancreatic cancer. *J. Pathol.* **166**, (1992) 7-12.

[22] Carraway KLIII, Cantley LC,. A neu acquaintance for erbB3 and erbB4: a role for receptor heterodimerization in growth signaling. *Cell* **78**, (1994) 5-8.

[23] Carpenter G, Cohen S,. Human epidermal growth factor and the proliferation of human firoblasts. *J. Cell Physiol.* **88**, (1976) 227-237.

[24] Ohlsson B, *et al.* Epidermal growth factor induces cell proliferation in mouse pancreas and salivary glands. *Pancreas* **14**, (1997) 94-98.

[25] Yamanaka Y, *et al.* Overexpression of HER2/neu oncogene in human pancreatic carcinoma. *Hum. Pathol.* **24**, (1997) 1127-1134.

[26] Barton CM, *et al.* Transforming growth factor alpha and epidermal growth factor in human pancreatic cancer. *J. Pathol.* **163**, (1991a) 111-116.
[27] Yamanaka Y, *et al.* Coexpression of epidermal growth factor receptor and ligands in human pancreatic cancer is associated with enhanced tumor aggressiveness. *Anticancer Res.* **13**, (1993b) 565-569.
[28] Ebert M, *et al.* Induction and expression of amphiregulin in human pancreatic cancer. *Cancer Res.* **54**, (1994a) 3959-3962.
[29] Yokoyama M, *et al.* Amphiregulin is a potent mitogen in human pancreatic cancer cells: correlation with patient survival. *Int. J. Oncol.* **6**, (1995) 625-631.
[30] Funatomi H, *et al.* Amphiregulin antisense oligonucleotide inhibits the growth of T3M4 human pancreatic cancer cells and sensitizes the cells to EGF receptor-targeted therapy. *Int. J. Cancer* **72**, (1997) 512-517.
[31] Yokoyama M, *et al.* Heparin-binding EGF-like growth factor expression and biological action in human pancreatic cancer cells. *Int. J. Oncol.* **8**, (1996) 289-295.
[32] Toyoda H, *et al.* Epiregulin: a novel epidermal growth factor with mitogenic activity for rat primary hepatocytes. *J. Biol. Chem.* **270**, (1995) 7495-7500.
[33] Hall PA, *et al.* The c-erbB-2 proto-oncogene in human pancreatic cancer. *J. Pathol.* **161**, (1990) 195-200.
[34] Lemoine NR, *et al.* The erbB-3 gene in human pancreatic cancer. *J. Pathol.* **168**, (1992) 269-273.
[35] Satoh K, *et al.* An immunohistochemical study of the c-erbB-2 oncogene product in intraductal mucin-hypersecreting neoplasms and in ductal cell carcinomas of the pancreas. *Cancer* **72**, (1993) 51-56.
[36] Dugan MC, *et al.* HER-2/neu expression in pancreatic adenocarcinoma: relation to tumor differentiation and survival. *Pancreas* **14**, (1997) 229-236.
[37] Friess H, *et al.* Enhanced erbB-3 expression in human pancreatic cancer correlates with tumour progression. *Clin. Cancer Res.* **1**, (1995) 1413-1420.
[38] Jiang WG, Hiscox S,. Hepatocyte growth factor/scatter factor, a cytokine playing multiple and converse roles. *Histol. Histopathol.* **12**, (1997) 537-555.
[39] Ebert M, *et al.* Coexpression of the c-met proto-oncogene and hepatocyte growth factor in human pancreatic cancer. *Cancer Res.* **54**, (1994b) 5775-5778.
[40] Di Renzo MF, *et al.* Expression of the Met/hepatocyte growth factor receptor in human pancreatic cancer. *Cancer Res.* **55**, (1995) 1129-1138.
[41] Furukawa T, *et al.* Hepatocyte growth factor and Met receptor expression in human pancreatic carcinogenesis. *Am. J. Pathol.* **147**, (1995) 889-895.
[42] Gold LI, Korc M,. Expression of transforming growth factor-β1, 2, and 3 mRNA and protein in human cancers. *Dig. Surg.* **11**, (1994) 150-156.
[43] van Laethem JL, *et al.* Different expression of transforming growth factor β_1 in pancreatic ductal adenocarcinoma and cystic neoplasms. *Pancreas* **15**, (1997) 41-47.

[44] Friess H, *et al.* Enhanced expression of the type II transforming growth factor beta receptor in human pancreatic cancer cells without alteration of type III receptor expression. *Cancer Res.* **53**, (1993) 2704-2707.
[45] Leung HY, Gullick WJ, Lemoine NR,. Expression and functional activity of fibroblast growth factors and their receptors in human pancreatic cancer. *Int. J. Cancer* **59**, (1994a) 667-675.
[46] Yamanaka Y, *et al.* Overexpression of acidic and basic fibroblast growth-factors in human pancreatic cancer correlates with advanced tumor stage. *Cancer Res.* **53**, (1993c) 5289-5296.
[47] Leung HY, *et al.* Localization of expression of fibroblast growth factors and their receptors in pancreatic adenocarcinoma by in-situ hybridization. *Int. J. Oncol.* **4**, (1994b) 1219-1223.
[48] Yamazaki K, *et al.* Expression of basic fibroblast growth factor (FGF-2)-associated with tumour proliferation in human pancreatic carcinoma. *Virchows Arch.* **431**, (1997) 95-101.
[49] Christofori G, Naik P, Hanahan D,. Vascular endothelial growth factor and its receptors, flt-1 and flk-1, are expressed in normal pancreatic islets and throughout islet cell tumorigenesis. *Mol. Endocrinol.* **9**, (1995) 1760-1770.
[50] Rooman I, Schuit F, Bouwens L,. Effect of vascular endothelial growth factor on growth and differentiation of pancreatic ductal epithelium. *Lab. Invest.* **76**, (1997) 225-232.
[51] Itakura J, *et al.* Enhanced expression of vascular endothelial growth factor in human pancreatic cancer correlates with local disease progression. *Clin. Cancer Res.* **3**, (1997) 1309-1316.
[52] Giguere V. Retinoic acid receptors and cellular retinoid binding proteins: complex interplay in retinoid signaling. *Endocr. Rev.* **15**, (1994) 61-79.
[53] Zugmaier G, *et al.* Growth-inhibitory effects of vitamin D analogues and retinoids on human pancreatic cancer cells. *Br. J. Cancer* **73**, (1996) 1341-1346.
[54] Rosewicz S, *et al.* Retinoids inhibit adhesion to laminin in human pancreatic carcinoma cells via the $\alpha_6\beta_1$-integrin receptor. *Gastroenterology* **112**, (1997) 532-542.

[55] Xu XC, *et al.* Differential suppression of nuclear retinoic acid receptor beta in pancreatic carcinomas. *Int. J. Oncol.* **8**, (1996) 445-451.

[56] Kaiser A, *et al.* Retinoic acid receptor β regulates growth and differentiation in human pancreatic carcinoma cells. *Gastroenterology* **113**, (1997) 920-929.

[57] Cheng JQ, *et al.* Amplification of AKT2 in human pancreatic cancer cells and inhibition of AKT2 expression and tumorigenicity by antisense RNA. *Proc. Natl. Acad. Sci. USA* **93**, (1996) 3636-3641.

[58] Barton CM, *et al.* Abnormalities of the p53 tumour suppressor gene in human pancreatic cancer. *Br. J. Cancer* **64**, (1991b) 1076-1082.

[59] Scarpa A, *et al.* Pancreatic adenocarcinomas frequently show p53 gene mutations. *Am. J. Pathol.* **142**, (1993) 1534-1543.

[60] Suwa H, *et al.* Clinical significance of serum p53 antigen in patients with pancreatic carcinomas. *Gut* **40**, (1997) 647-653.

[61] Luo JC, *et al.* Levels of p53 antigen in the plasma of patients with adenomas and carcinomas of the colon. *Cancer Lett.* **91**, (1995) 235-240.

[62] Fontanini G, *et al.* Levels of p53 antigen in the serum of non-small lung cancer patients correlate with positive p53 immunohistochemistry on tumor sections, tumor necrosis and nodal involvement. *Int. J. Oncol.* **5**, (1994) 553-558.

[63] Rozenblum E, *et al.* Tumor-suppressive pathways in pancreatic carcinoma. *Cancer Res.* **57**, (1997) 1731-1734.

[64] Schutte M, *et al.* Abrogation of the Rb/p16 tumor-suppressive pathway in virtually all pancreatic carcinomas. *Cancer Res.* **57**, (1997) 3126-3130.

[65] Hussussian CJ, *et al.* Germline p16 mutations in familial melanoma. *Nat. Genet.* **8**, (1994) 15-21.

[66] Nobori T, *et al.* Deletions of the cyclin-dependent kinase-4 inhibitor gene in multiple human cancers. *Nature* **368**, (1994) 753-756.

[67] Quelle DE, *et al.* Alternative reading frames of the INK4a tumor suppressor gene encode two unrelated proteins capable of inducing cell cycle arrest. *Cell* **83**, (1995) 993-1000.

[68] Zhang Y, Xiong Y, Yarbrough WG,. (1998) ARF promotes MDM2 degradation and stabilizes p53: ARF-INK4a locus deletion impairs both the Rb and p53 tumor suppression pathways. *Cell* **92**, 725-734.

[69] Naumann M, *et al.* Frequent codeletion of p16/MTS1 and p15/MTS2 and genetic alterations in p16/MTS1 in pancreatic tumors. *Gastroenterology* **110**, (1996) 1215-1224.

[70] Schutte M, *et al.* DPC4 gene in various tumor types. *Cancer Res.* **56**, (1996) 2527-2530.

[71] de Winter JP, *et al.* DPC4 (SMAD4) mediates transforming growth factor-β1 (TGF-β1) induced growth inhibition and transcriptional response in breast tumour cells. *Oncogene* **14**, (1997) 1891-1899.

[72] Liu F, *et al.* A human Mad protein acting as a BMP-regulated transcriptional activator. *Nature* **381**, (1996) 620-623.

[73] Hahn SA, *et al.* DPC4, a candidate tumor suppressor gene at human chromosome 18q21.1. *Science* **271**, (1996) 350-353.

[74] Moskaluk CA, *et al.* Genomic sequencing of DPC4 in the analysis of familial pancreatic carcinoma. *Diagn. Mol. Pathol.* **6**, (1997b) 85-90.

[75] Bartsch D, *et al.* Mutations of the DPC4/Smad4 gene in neuroendocrine pancreatic tumors. *Oncogene* **18**, (1999) 2367-2371.

[76] Barton CM, *et al.* Abnormalities of the RB1 and DCC tumor suppressor genes: uncommon in human pancreatic adenocarcinoma. *Mol. Carcinog.* **13**, (1995) 61-69.

[77] Goggins M, *et al.* Germline BRCA2 gene mutations in patients with apparently sporadic pancreatic carcinomas. *Cancer Res.* **56**, (1996) 5360-5364.

[78] Su GH, *et al.* Germline and somatic mutations of the STK11/LKB1 Peutz-Jeghers gene in pancreatic and biliary cancers. *Am. J. Pathol.* **154**, (1999) 1835-1840.

[79] Hiyama E, *et al.* Telomerase activity is detected in pancreatic cancer but not in benign tumors. *Cancer Res.* **57**, (1997) 326-331.

[80] Hahn SA, *et al.* Alleotype of pancreatic adenocarcinoma using xenograft enrichment. *Cancer Res.* **55**, (1995) 4670-4675.

[81] Emmert-Buck MR, *et al.* Laser capture microdissection. *Science* **274**, 998-1001.

[82] Lisitsyn N, Lisitsina N, Wigler M,. Cloning the differences between two complex genomes. *Science* **259**, (1993) 946-951.

[83] Schutte M, *et al.* Identification by representational difference analysis of a homozygous deletion in pancreatic carcinoma that lies within the BRCA2 region. *Proc. Natl. Acad. Sci. USA* **92**, (1995) 5950-5954.

Part I: Genetic alterations in pancreatic cancer

Molecular Pathogenesis of Pancreatic Cancer
T.M. Gress (Ed.)
IOS Press, 2000

Genomic RDA for the identification of chromosomal aberrations in pancreatic cancer: merits and drawbacks

C. Wallrapp[1], S. Hähnel[1], C. Sorio[2], A. Scarpa[2], T.M. Gress[1]
1) Department of Internal Medizin I, Universitätsklinikum Ulm, 89081 Ulm, Germany
2) Dipartimento di Patologia - Anatomia Patologica, Università di Verona, I-37134 Verona, Italy

The identification of novel tumour suppressor loci is often led by the detection of regions recurrently deleted in tumours [1]. In contrast overrepresentations of DNA, and in particular high level amplifications may lead to the identification of protooncogenes [2, 3]. Various methods are currently available for the identification of genomic imbalances. *C*omparative *G*enomic *H*ybridisation (CGH) is frequently used for a genome wide analysis of chromosomal aberrations [4, 5]. In a recent CGH analysis of pancreatic adenocarcinoma we could show the most common overrepresentations on chromosomes 16p, 20q, 22q, and 17q and underrepresentations on a subregion of chromosome 9p. Distinct high-level amplifications were found on 1p32-p34, 6q24, 7q22, 12p13 and 22q [2]. While the characterisation of deletions identified by CGH proofed difficult since deleted areas have to exceed 10 Mb in size in order to be detectable [6], characterisation of high-level amplifications usually confined to DNA segments < 1 Mb was more successful. In this context the *c-myb* protoncogene was identified as the relevant gene involved in a high-level amplification on 6q23-24 [3].

A more advanced scheme for identification of genomic alterations, named representational difference analysis (RDA), was introduced by Lisitsyn et al. [7]. This PCR based technique takes advantage of reiterated subtractive and kinetic enrichment to isolate restriction endonuclease digested fragments present in one population of DNA fragments *(tester)* but not in another *(driver)*. In a first step, representations of the genomes that are to be compared are produced by adaptor-mediated PCR of restriction endonuclease digested fragments. Because of preferential amplification of smaller fragments, the resulting amplicons represent only a subset of the genome they originate from. The reduced complexity of the amplicons facilitates subtractive hybridization thus resulting in a more efficient enrichment of differences.

In the present project we used RDA to identify chromosomal areas deleted or amplified in pancreatic cancer. In the first phase of the project our major effort concentrated on the optimization of the RDA-protocol for the use with human pancreatic cancer samples. Naturally, surgical specimens are not suitable for this purpose due to the small number of tumour cells (at most 10-20%) usually present in pancreatic cancer tissues. Therefore, enrichment techniques as e.g. microdissection have to be used. In our hands microdissected material from paraffin embedded specimens was not suitable for RDA analyses as it repeatedly failed to generate *bona fide* difference products. It has to be assumed that random strand breakages induced by formaldehyde fixation are responsible for this failure. Nude mouse xenografts of pancreatic cancer tissues have been successfully used by the Johns Hopkins group to identify the BRCA2 region in pancreatic cancer [8].

However, even when using xenografted tissues several difficulties were evident. Ideally expanded tumour cells should make up to 50% of the xenograft mass to ensure the reliable identification of amplifications. Even so nude mouse DNA must be added to the *driver* to avoid the selection of mouse sequences, which are of course present in the xenograft only. The fraction of tumour cells must exceed 50% of the xenograft mass to allow the identification of deletions. Even so it is a prerequisite, that no normal human cells are retained and the stroma of the xenograft is made up of mouse tissue only. The choice of the appropriate *tester/driver* source is as well of importance. Ideally *tester* and *driver* DNA should be derived from the same type of source and should be extracted with the same technique. In our hands the use of DNA extracted from peripheral blood as *tester* (for deletions) or *driver* (for amplifications) was not successful. DNA extracted from peripheral blood is of a different quality than the DNA extracted from snap frozen tissue blocks. In general DNA from peripheral blood is of higher molecular weight and more difficult to restriction digest to completion than DNA from tissue blocks. These differences in DNA quality due to the extraction procedure and the source will generate artificial differences between *tester* and *driver* and thus lead to spurious results. In the same way it is important to check the quality of undigested DNA on an agarose gel prior to the start of the RDA-protocol. It has to be ensured that the quality is similar between *tester* and *driver*. RDA will predominantely detect the most abundant and largest deletion occurring in a certain tumour. To avoid selecting fragments from the major known deletions in pancreatic cancer (9p, 17p, 18q) one should attempt to use tissue samples ideally tested to be devoid of one or more of the known deletions. This is certainly a condition that is almost impossible to achieve, but it should be kept in mind when selecting tissue samples for RDA. Once the RDA-protocol has started it usually takes many hours of painful work to find out, that the experiment failed due to the wrong selection of *tester* or *driver*, or that once again one has succeeded in identifying the 9p deletion. In this context we would as well strongly recommend to use only DNA from female patients when searching for deletions. This recommendation is based on the results of a recent RDA experiment designed to identify DNA-fragments deleted in pancreatic cancer by subtracting DNA derived from a xenograft of pancreatic carcinoma tissue (the *driver*) from the corresponding normal DNA of a male caucasian patient (the *tester*). This was one of the most successful approaches and yielded 10 *bona fide* differential bands. Southern blot hybridizations revealed that 3 of these fragments were apparently homozygously deleted and 7 heterozygously deleted in the primary tumour used for the RDA experiment (Figure 1).

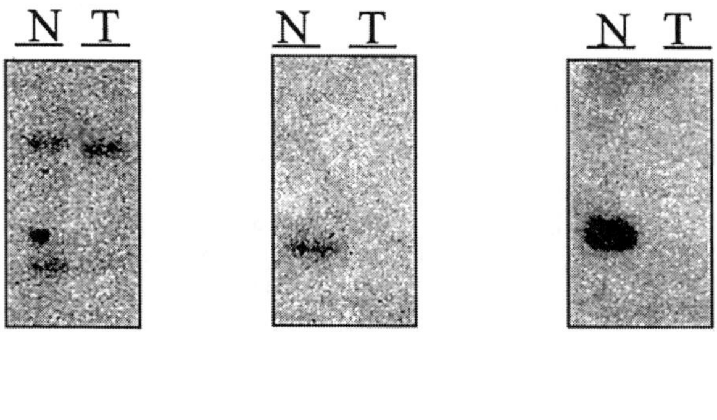

Figure 1:
Southern Blots with 5µg *Bgl*II digested tester and driver DNA used in this RDA experiment., (N: DNA from normal tissue; T: DNA from a pancreatic cancer xenograft)

Hybridizations with Southern blots containing DNA of pancreatic cancer cell lines, revealed that 2 of the isolated fragments appeared to be homozygously deleted in 10/15 pancreatic cancer cell lines. (Figure 2).

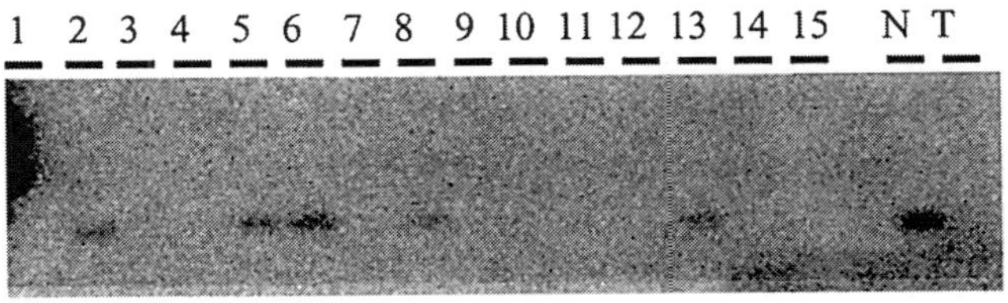

Figure 2:
1-15: 5 µg *BglII* digested DNA from pancreatic cancer cell lines. N: 5µg BglII digested DNA from normal tissue used as *tester* and T: BglII digested DNA tumour tisue used as *driver*.

However, it turned out that these two fragments originated from the Y-chromosome, and that fragments of the Y-chromosome were deleted in virtually all cell lines of male origin. Loss of the Y chromosome is a common feature in many tumours [9]. Whether loss of the Y chromosome is of functional significance in neoplastic cells is unknown at present. Though loss of the Y chromosome is probably not a rate limiting step in cancerogenesis it is a consistent chromosomal imbalance in pancreatic cancer occurring frequently *in vitro* in cell lines and *in vivo* in xenografts of male origin These results led to our recommendation not to use DNA from male pancreatic cancer patients for RDA approaches. Usually large fragments or the entire Y-chromosome are absent in pancreatic cancer tissues, which will lead to a predominant selection of RDA fragments from the Y-chromosome.

To summarize, in our hands RDA is a highly efficient technique to identify genomic alterations in tumours, with the major advantage of directly obtaining DNA fragments from the deleted or amplified area for further analyses e.g. to isolate YAC or BAC clones. However, the technology is not trivial and many issues have to be considered before starting an RDA approach.
The major issues that proved of relevance in our hands are summarized in table 1.

Table 1: „Ideal“ starting material for RDA:

- **Deletions:**
  Tester: normal pancreas (no DNA from peripheral blood)
  Driver: Xenografts with > 50% tumour cell enrichment
  (no primary tumour no microdissected tissue)
- **Amplifications:**
  Tester: Xenografts with 30-50% tumour cell enrichment (see above)
  Driver: normal pancreas+nude mouse DNA (e.g. liver, pancreas)
- Use tester/driver DNA of a similar quality
- Use tumours with the smallest number of major known deletions
- Use tumours from female patients

Acknowledgements

This work was supported in part by grants from the European Union (BMH4-CT98-3085) and the German Ministery for Education and Research (BMBF:GB9401) to TMG.

Literature

[1] E.R. Fearon, Human cancer syndromes: clues to the origin and nature of cancer Science **278** (1997) 1043-1050.

[2] S.Solinas Toldo *et al*, Mapping of chromosomal imbalances in pancreatic carcinoma by comparative genomic hybridization. Cancer Res **56** (1996), 3803-3807.

[3] C.Wallrapp *et al*, Characterization of a high copy number amplification at 6q24 in pancreatic cancer identifies c-*myb* as a candidate oncogene. Cancer Res **57** (1997) 3135-3139.

[4] M.Nessling M. *et al*, Mapping of chromosomal imbalances in gastric adenocarcinoma revealed amplified protooncogenes MYCN, MET, WNT2, and ERBB2. Genes Chromosom. Cancer **23** (1999) 307-316.

[5] S. du Manoir *et al*, Detection of complete and partial chromosome gains and losses by comparative genomic in situ hybridization. Hum Genet 90 (1993), 590-610.

[6] M.Bentz *et al*, Minimal sizes of deletions detected by comparative genomic hybridization. Genes Chromosom.Cancer.**21** (1998) 172-175.

[7] N.Lisitsyn *et al*, Cloning the differences between two complex genomes. Science **259** (1993) 946-951.

[8] M. Schutte *et al*., Identification by representational difference analysis of a homozygous deletion in pancreatic cancer that lies within the BRCA2 region Proc. Natl Acad. Sci. USA, **92** (1995) 5950-5954.

[9] S. Hunter *et al*, Y chromosome loss in esophageal carcinoma: an in situ hybridization study. Genes Chromosomes Cancer. **8** (1993) 172-177.

Molecular Pathogenesis of Pancreatic Cancer
T.M. Gress (Ed.)
IOS Press, 2000

Chromosomal imbalances in pancreatic tumors detected by arbitrarily primed PCR Fingerprinting

A. Scarpa, M. Scardoni, G. Rigaud, P. Moore and G. Zamboni

Pathology Department, Section of Anatomical Pathology, Università di Verona, Italy

Little or no information is known about the chromosomal and molecular abnormalities in pancreatic neoplasms other than common ductal cancer. These tumor entities comprise those arising from both the exocrine and endocrine pancreas. The study of these less common tumor types should lead not only to a greater understanding of the genetic events leading to their pathogenesis, but will also provide an answer to the question of whether or not similar biochemical pathways are responsible for neoplastic transformation and progression of different pancreatic malignancies.

Arbitrarily primed polymerase chain reaction (AP-PCR) is a DNA fingerprinting technique used to detect chromosomal abnormalities [1, 2, 4-6]. Using single primers which anneal at multiple sites, many PCR products are generated providing a distinct DNA fingerprint. Comparison of AP-PCR fingerprints generated from tumor DNA with those from matched normal DNA allows the detection of qualitative and quantitative changes occurring at individual loci. Decreased intensity of AP-PCR bands in tumor tissue reflects allelic losses, whereas increased band intensity in tumor DNA reflects an increase in copy number. Furthermore, the chromosomal origins of these fingerprint bands may be assigned by concomitant AP-PCR of somatic monochromosome cell hybrid panels [1, 2, 11].

We have used AP-PCR fingerprinting obtained with two arbitrary primers to identify chromosomal imbalances in various types of pancreatic cancer. In particular, we analyzed 30 cases of ductal cancer, 10 cases of intraductal papillary mucinous tumors, 6 cases of solid papillary tumors, 5 cases of acinar carcinoma and 20 ampullary tumors. The arbitrary primers used were MCG1 and AR3 [2, 6].

Examples of the AP-PCR fingerprints generated are shown in Figure 1, where specific alterations in copy number of individual loci can be visualized. The chromosomal location of these different bands is also indicated. Two arbitrary primers yielded a total of 45 fingerprint bands, 21 from MCG1 and 24 from AR-3 fingerprints with determined chromosomal location. Eighteen chromosomes were represented by at least one fingerprint band, although the number of bands originating from each chromosome varied. Chromosome 7 was represented by five bands, chromosomes 2, 3 and X by four bands and the remaining chromosomes by three bands or less. Chromosomes 10, 14, 18, 19 and 21 were not represented by distinct fingerprint bands. The status of these individual bands was then compiled for each case and subsequently grouped together to obtain an AP-PCR amplotype generated for each tumor type. The results of the analysis are summarized in Table 1. Nonrandom chromosomal imbalances were considered as those occurring in at least 30% of cases and detected by the same AP-PCR fingerprint band.

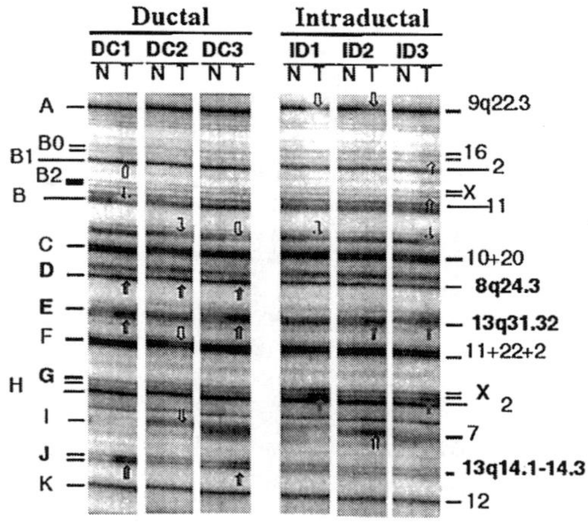

Figure 1. Example of AP-PCR fingerprints ductal cancer and intraductal tumors using MCG1 arbitrary primer. Case number is reported on the top, where N and T indicate the lanes containing matched normal and tumor DNA, respectively. The bands composing the fingerprints are indicated by letters to the left, while their chromosomal origin is indicated to the right. The arrows indicate selected bands showing an increased (upward arrows) or decreased (downward arrows) intensity in tumor with respect to normal DNA, after subtraction of background.

Table 1. Nonrandom chromosomal imbalances detected in various tumor types

Tumor type	% cases	GAIN	LOSS
Ductal cancer	>50	1q, 8q, 9q 13q14-q31	5, 7, 9, 10, 17
Intraductal tumors	>30	1q, X	9q
Ampullary tumors	>30	1, 7, 9, X, 13q14-q31	3, 5, 9, 10, 17
Acinar cancer	>50	2, 12, X	16
Solid-papillary tumors	>30	20	-

The validity of our AP-PCR data is substantiated by: i) the ability of AP-PCR to detect moderate changes in chromosomal copy number, as clearly demonstrated by the unequivocal determination of subject gender by the intensity of AP-PCR bands originating from chromosome X [9]; and ii) the analysis of acinar carcinomas by comparative genomic hybridization (CGH) technique, which confirmed the nonrandom losses on chromosome 16 and gains on chromosomes 12 and X [10]. In addition, our allelotype analysis on the consensus regions of gain or loss in this latter tumor type showed allelic imbalances consistent with the CGH profiles in most cases (Figure 2).

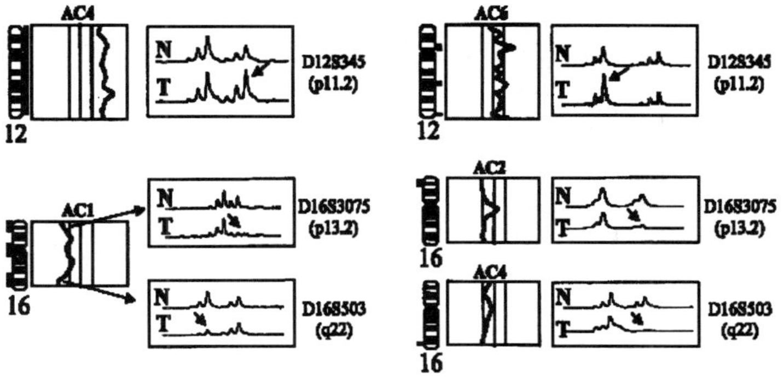

Figure 2. Representative CGH profiles and DNA microsatellite analysis of selected chromosomal loci. Bars on the left and on the right of each chromosome indicate losses and gains, respectively. The case number is indicated on the top of each CGH profile. The profiles show the mean tumor to normal fluorescence ratio along the chromosomes. The line in the middle of the profiles indicates the base line ratio (1.0), the left and the right lines indicate ratio values of 0.75 and 1.25, taken as the threshold limits for chromosomal losses and gains, respectively. On the right of each CGH profile are shown the electropherogram tracings of microsatellite analysis for the loci indicated, whose chromosomal location is reported in parenthesis. The upper and lower curves correspond to the electrophoretic tracings of normal (N) and tumor (T) DNA. The arrows indicate the allele showing higher intensity signal or loss in tumor DNA with respect to the matched normal allele.

CONCLUSIONS

The molecular karyotype of the different exocrine pancreatic tumors using two arbitrary primers indicates that each pancreatic tumor type shows a characteristic pattern of chromosomal alterations. This therefore suggests that the biochemical pathways involved in exocrine pancreatic tumorigenesis is distinct according to histologic type of neoplasia.

One intriguing piece of information is the finding of nonrandom amplification on chromosome X common to a proportion of ampullary, intraductal and acinar tumors. Gains of Xq have been seen in different B-cell lymphoma types, with a reported frequency of about 30% [3, 9]. Among solid tumors, only four out of 27 tumor types studied showed amplifications on Xq in at least 20% of cases, including prostatic, testicular, cervical and non-functioning pituitary tumors. Among the remaining 23 tumor types, only breast and brain cancers showed Xq amplifications in at least 10% of cases [8]. A candidate oncogene has been recently identified on Xq22-24 [7] and its involvement in ampullary and acinar cancers is under evaluation.

The AP-PCR analysis also gives further insight into the nature of chromosomal anomalies. In many instances, AP-PCR detected coexistent gains and and losses on the same chromosome, suggesting that these imbalances may be a consequence of more complex phenomena, such as unbalanced translocations or other chromosomal rearrangements. In addition, comparison between AP-PCR and CGH suggests that anomalies affecting the same chromosomal regions may occur at much higher frequencies than expected, suggesting that genomic amplifications are usually confined to DNA segments smaller than the megabase long segments required for detection in CGH. Modest increases in genetic material may be as effective as higher level amplifications when affecting sites where a proto-oncogene resides.

Additional arbitrary primers are being used to obtain a more detailed analysis of the chromosomal imbalances occuring in pancreatic tumors.

Acknowledgements

Supported by grants from Consorzio Studi Universitari di Verona, Italy; the Associazione Italiana Ricerca Cancro (AIRC) to A.S., Milan, Italy; cofinanced grant from Verona University and Ministero Università e Ricerca Scientifica e Tecnologica (MURST, COFIN 9806151968_002 - COFIN 9906218982_003), Rome, Italy; and European Community grant BIOMED 2 CE-Contract No. BMH4-CT98-3805.

Literature

[1] A. Achille, *et al.*, Chromosome 5 allelic losses are early events in tumors of the papilla of Vater and occur at sites similar to those of gastric cancer. Br J Cancer **78** (1998), 1653-1660.

[2] A. Achille, *et al.*, Chromosome 7q allelic losses in pancreatic carcinoma. Cancer Res **56** (1996), 3808-3813.

[3] D.W. Hammond, *et al.*, Cytogenetic analysis of a United Kingdom series of non-Hodgkins lymphomas. Cancer Genet Cytogenet **61** (1992), 31-38.

[4] Y. Ionov, *et al.*, Ubiquitous somatic mutations in simple repeated sequences reveal a new mechanism for colonic carcinogenesis. Nature **363** (1993), 558-561.

[5] S. Malkhosyan, *et al.*, Molecular karyotype (amplotype) of metastatic colorectal cancer by unbiased arbitrarily primed PCR DNA fingerprinting. Proc Natl Acad Sci USA **95** (1998), 10170-10175.

[6] M.A. Peinado, *et al.*, Isolation and characterization of allelic losses and gains in colorectal tumors by arbitrary primed polymerase chain reaction. Proc Natl Acad Sci USA **89** (1992), 10065-10069.

[7] M. Prosniak, *et al.*, A novel candidate oncogene, MCT-1, is involved in cell cycle progression. Cancer Res **58** (1998), 4233-4237.

[8] P.H. Rooney, *et al.*, Comparative genomic hybridization and chromosomal instability in solid tumours. Br J Cancer **80** (1999), 862-873.

[9] A. Scarpa, *et al.*, Non-random chromosomal imbalances in primary mediastinal B-cell lymphoma detected by arbitrarily primed PCR fingerprinting. Genes Chromosomes Cancer **26** (1999), 203-209.

[10] D. Taruscio, *et al.*, Pancreatic acinar carcinoma shows a distinct pattern of chromosomal imbalances by comparative genomic hybridization. Genes Chromosom Cancer **in press** (2000).

[11] J. Yasuda, *et al.*, Chromosomal assignment of human DNA fingerprint sequences by simultaneous hybridization to arbitrarily primed PCR products from human/rodent monochromosome cell hybrids. Genomics **34** (1996), 1-8.

Genome-Wide Allelotyping of Pancreatic Acinar Cell and Nonfunctional Endocrine Tumors

Gildas Rigaud, Giuseppe Zamboni, Patrick S. Moore, Massimo Falconi, Aldo Scarpa
Pathology Department, Section of Anatomical Pathology (G.R., G.Z, P.S.M., A.S.) and Surgery Department (M.F.) Università di Verona, Italy

Pancreatic acinar cell (PAC) and nonfunctional endocrine tumors (NF-PETs) are uncommon neoplasms for which little information is available regarding the chromosomal and molecular alterations giving rise to malignancy. In the former tumors, no aberrations have been found in the four genes most frequently altered in pancreatic ductal cancers, namely K-*ras*, *p53*, *p16* and *DPC4* [3, 8, 12]. In NF-PET, it is clear that neither K-*ras* nor *p53* have any significant role in tumorigenesis, while alteration of the *p16* and *DPC4* genes have been reported to be frequent events [1, 6] in spite of the fact that allelic losses on chromosomes 9p and 18q are infrequent in these tumors [3].

As PAC may express neuroendocrine markers and mixed exocrine and endocrine pancreatic cancers exist [7, 11], one interesting question is whether PET shares molecular events with acinar or ductal carcinoma (PDC). This is also relevant in the light of recent reports suggesting that a proportion of PET show anomalies in *p16/MTS1* and *DPC4/Smad4* genes which are frequently altered in pancreatic ductal cancer [1, 6], thus suggesting that common genetic anomalies may underlie the transformation of a pancreatic stem cell from which the different pancreatic tumor types arise.

The identification of commonly deleted chromosomal regions by loss of heterozygosity (LOH) analysis using PCR amplification of polymorphic microsatellite repeats in tumor and matched normal DNA and may aid in the localization of tumor suppressor genes. When this analysis is extended to multiple chromosomal arms a distinct allelotype is generated. No such data is available for PAC due to their rarity. The only allelotype study available for PET suggested that these tumors are characterized by a low frequency of chromosomal allelic deletions and was based on the analysis of seven NF-PETs using two markers per chromosomal arm [4]. Here we report a high resolution allelotype for both PAC and NF-PET obtained by the use of 394 microsatellite markers covering all 22 autosomes.

Generation of an allelotype for PAC

Five cases for which DNA from frozen tissue was available were analyzed using 394 microsatellite markers. The results are shown in Figure 3. Chromosomes 1p, 4q and 17p showed LOH in >70% of cases and chromosomes 11q, 13q, 15q and 16q in 60-70% of cases. Chromosomes 3q, 6q, 8q, 18q and 21q showed losses in 50-60% of cases. All the remaining chromosomes showed no or few allelic losses. Putative smallest common deleted regions were localized at 1p36.31, 3p25.2, 4q26-31.1, 15q15.1-22.1 and 16q21.1-q22.1. The resulting allelotype of PAC is markedly different from that of either ductal or endocrine tumors of the pancreas and the involvement of chromosome 4q and 16q seems characteristic of this tumor type.

High resolution allelotype of nonfunctional PET

Each of 16 NF-PET for which DNA from frozen tissue was available was analyzed for allelic loss at 394 microsatellite loci. Representative results are shown in Figure 1. The comprehensive allelotype is shown in Figure 2. Frequent LOH was found on chromosome arms 6q and 11q in greater than 60% of cases, while about 50% of cases had losses on 11p, 20q and 21. Chromosomes 2p and 10p showed loss in 44%, while the remaining chromosome arms had allelic losses in less than 40% of cases.

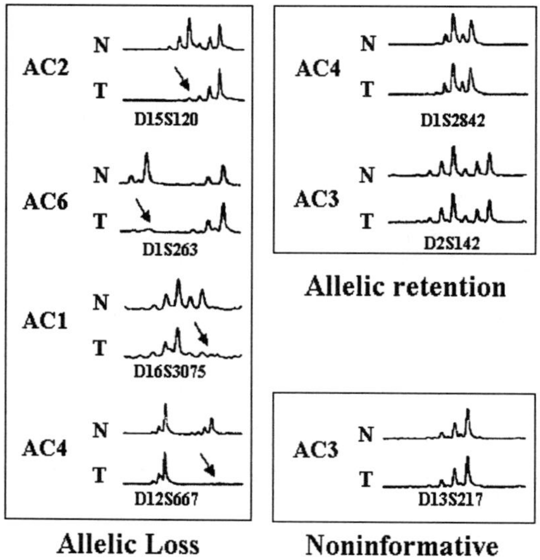

Figure 1. Representative electropherogram tracings of microsatellite analysis. Loci and case numbers are as indicated along with examples showing allelic loss, retention and a noninformative locus. N, normal; T, tumor.

Overlapping of the interstitial allelic deletions localized two putative smallest common deleted regions (SCDR) were localized at chromosome bands 6q22.1 and 11q22.1. The average fractional allelic loss (FAL) was 0.33, calculated as the number of chromosomal arms having allelic loss divided by the total number of informative chromosomal arms. However, the contribution to the total FAL was mainly due to seven cases showing more than 10 chromosomal arms affected by deletions with a mean FAL of 0.55. The remaining nine cases showing less than 10 arms with allelic loss and had a mean FAL of 0.15. Thus NF-PET may be divided in two groups, one showing a high degree of large chromosomal allelic deletions, and a second with a low number of scattered losses with no apparent specific localization.

Conclusions

PAC displays a relatively high degree of allelic loss on several chromosomes with a mean FAL of 0.33. Chromosome arms 1p, 4q, 11q, 13q, 15q, 16q and 17p show a high frequency of allelic loss. identified SCDRs on chromosomes 1p36.31, 3p25.2, 4q26-31.1, 15q15.1-22.1 and 16q21.1-q22.1. In PAC, losses on chromosomes 9p and 18q were relatively infrequent and no alterations in either *p16* or *Smad4* are found (Moore, et al.). The SCDR at 3p25.2 in PAC is telomeric to the *FHIT* gene, located at 3p14.2, that has recently been implicated in PDC [10]. Although the *VHL* gene maps to 3p25-26 and is altered in a subset of sporadic pancreatic serous cystadenomas [13], no mutations in were detected by either single strand conformation polymorphism or direct sequence analysis (data not shown).

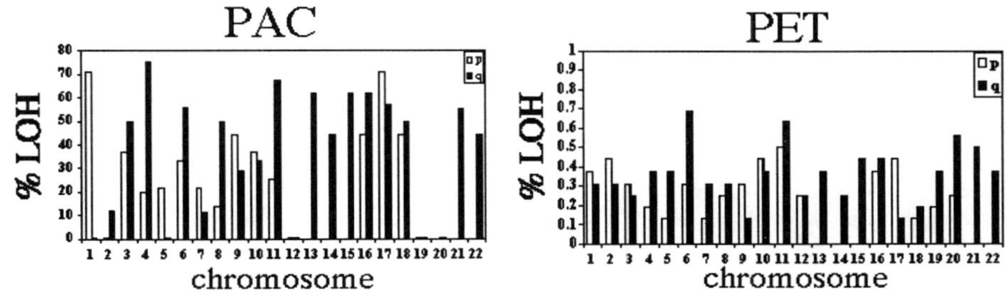

Figure 2. Allelotype of PAC and PET.

The apparent division of NF-PETs into two subgroups based on differences in the frequency and type of allelic losses is of particular interest, although no perceptible correlations were evident between these subgroups and clinical parameters. The losses in the low-FAL subgroup were not localized to any particular region. The existence of two molecular phenotypes among PETs can however be inferred by reports on the ploidy pattern of these tumors and by a recent study using comparative genomic hybridization (CGH) [11].

In NF-PETs, genetic losses involving chromosome 11q were highly frequent. The *MEN1* gene is located on this chromosome and is obviously involved in the familial syndrome. However, a proportion of sporadic NF-PET also have somatic mutations of this gene [2, 5]. Our high resolution allelotype study localized a putative SCDR to band 11q22.1, which is distal to the *MEN1* gene located at 11q13. This, together with the large losses observed which involve the entire chromosome, is suggestive that there are additional tumor suppressor genes reside on chromosome 11.

Chromosomal losses at 9p and 18q were not frequent events in NF-PETs. Given the recent reports of high frequencies of alterations in NF-PETs of the *p16* and *DPC4* genes [2, 5], a higher frequency of LOH would be expected if they are indeed involved in PET pathogenesis. Furthermore, we found no alterations in either *p16* or *DPC4* in 30 NF-PETs (see Moore, et al.). Taken together, this data suggests that these two genes are not likely to play a significant role in NF-PET pathogenesis.

The SCDR 1p36 in both PAC and PET encompasses the same region in which frequent LOH is present in PDC [9]. Although, chromosomal deletions at 1p36 are common events in a wide variety of tumor types, a target gene for this chromosomal region has yet to be identified. PDC is also characterized by highly frequent losses at chromosomes 9p, 17p and 18q [9], which with one exception are not implicated in either PAC or PET. Even though LOH on 17p may be a common event in PAC, the target of these losses is not the *p53* gene, as for PDC. The combination of chromosomal anomalies found by our extensive allelotyping substantiates the supposition that PDC, PAC, and PETs are each separate entities with distinct molecular mechanisms.

Acknowledgements

This study was supported by grants from Consorzio Studi Universitari di Verona, Italy; the Associazione Italiana Ricerca Cancro (AIRC) to A.S., Milan, Italy; cofinanced grant from Verona University and Ministero Università e Ricerca Scientifica e Tecnologica (MURST, COFIN 9806151968_002 - COFIN 9906218982_003), Rome, Italy; and European Community grant BIOMED 2 CE-Contract No. BMH4-CT98-3805.

Literature

[1] D. Bartsch, *et al.*, Mutations of the DPC4/Smad4 gene in neuroendocrine pancreatic tumors. Oncogene **18** (1999), 2367-2371.

[2] J.H. Bassett, *et al.*, Characterization of mutations in patients with multiple endocrine neoplasia type 1. Am J Hum Genet **62** (1998), 232-244.

[3] S. Beghelli, *et al.*, Pancreatic endocrine tumours: evidence for a tumour suppressor pathogenesis and for a tumour suppressor gene on chromosome 17p. J Pathol **186** (1998), 41-50.

[4] D.C. Chung, *et al.*, Localization of putative tumor suppressor loci by genome-wide allelotyping in human pancreatic endocrine tumors. Cancer Res **58** (1998), 3706-3711.

[5] O. Hessman, *et al.*, Mutation of the multiple endocrine neoplasia type 1 gene in nonfamilial, malignant tumors of the endocrine pancreas. Cancer Res **58** (1998), 377-379.

[6] P. Muscarella, *et al.*, Genetic alterations in gastrinomas and nonfunctioning pancreatic neuroendocrine tumors: an analysis of p16/MTS1 tumor suppressor gene inactivation. Cancer Res **58** (1998), 237-240.

[7] G. Rindi, *et al.*, Cell biology, clinicopathological profile, and classification of gastro- enteropancreatic endocrine tumors. J Mol Med **76** (1998), 413-420.

[8] E. Rozenblum, *et al.*, Tumor-suppressive pathways in pancreatic carcinoma. Cancer Res **57** (1997), 1731-1734.

[9] A.B. Seymour, *et al.*, Allelotype of pancreatic adenocarcinoma. Cancer Res **54** (1994), 2761-2764.

[10] C. Sorio, *et al.*, The FHIT gene is expressed in pancreatic ductular cells and is altered in pancreatic cancers. Cancer Res **59** (1999), 1308-1314.

[11] E.J. Speel, *et al.*, Genetic Differences in Endocrine Pancreatic Tumor Subtypes Detected by Comparative Genomic Hybridization. Am J Pathol **155** (1999), 1787-1794.

[12] P.G. Terhune, *et al.*, Only wild-type c-Ki-ras codons 12, 13, and 61 in human pancreatic acinar cell carcinomas. Mol Carcinog **10** (1994), 110-114.

[13] A.O. Vortmeyer, *et al.*, Allelic deletion and mutation of the von Hippel-Lindau (VHL) tumor suppressor gene in pancreatic microcystic adenomas. Am J Pathol **151** (1997), 951-956.

Mutations of the *DPC4/Smad4* Gene in Neuroendocrine Pancreatic Tumors

Detlef Bartsch[1], Stephan A. Hahn[2]
[1]*Departments of Surgery, Philipps-University Marburg, 35043 Marburg, Germany*
[2]*Department of Internal Medicine, University of Bochum, 44892 Bochum, Germany*

Abstract. Tumors of the endocrine pancreas are extremely rare, and molecular mechanisms leading to their development are not well understood. A candidate tumor suppressor gene, *DPC4*, located at 18q21, has recently been shown to be inactivated in half of pancreatic adenocarcinoma xenografts. The close anatomical relationship of the exocrine and endocrine pancreas prompted us to determine the role of *DPC4* in the tumorigenesis of 25 pancreatic islet cell tumors (11 insulinomas, 9 non-functioning endocrine carcinomas, 3 gastrinomas, 2 vipomas). A mutation screening of the highly conserved COOH-terminal domain of *DPC4* (exons 8 to 11) was performed by single-strand conformational variant analysis and a PCR-based deletion assay. Five of 9 (55%) non-functioning endocrine pancreatic carcinomas revealed either point mutations, small intragenic deletions or homozygous deletion of *DPC4* sequences compared to none of the insulinomas, gastrinomas or vipomas. These results suggest that *DPC4* is an important target gene promoting tumorigenesis of non-functioning neuroendocrine pancreatic carcinomas.

1. Introduction

Neuroendocrine pancreatic tumors (NPT) arise from the pancreatic islet cells and belong to the APUD (amine and precursor uptake and decarboxylation) system. These tumors are rare and account only for 1-5% of pancreatic tumors. About 90% of NPTs are characterized by the extensive production of polypeptide hormones, whereas the remaining 10% are non-functioning neuronedocrine neoplasms [1]. The most common NPT's are insulinomas and gastrinomas representing approximately 70% and 20% of NPT's, respectively. Vipomas, glucagonomas, somatostatinomas and others are extremely rare. Approximately 10% to 20% of NPT`s are associated with the multiple endocrine neoplasia type 1 (MEN1), an autosomal dominant inherited tumor syndrome that predisposes to develop NPTs [2].

Not least due to the rare occurrence of NPTs our knowledge of the genetic changes associated with the initiation and progression of these tumors is very limited, and available genetic data relys usually on small numbers of tumors analyzed. A considerably high number of genetic alterations were found in the recently cloned *Menin* gene at chromosome 11q13 which is responsible for the MEN1 syndrome [3]. Loss of heterozygosity including the region of the *Menin* gene was found in 93% of sporadic gastrinomas and in 50% of sporadic insulinomas. Somatic mutations of the M*enin* gene were identified in 33% of sporadic gastrinomas and 17% of sporadic insulinomas [4]. Amplification of *HER-2/neu* proto-oncogene was frequently observed in gastrinomas [5]. Furthermore, inactivation of the *p16*^{INK4a} tumor suppressor gene by either hypermethylation or homozygous deletion was identified in more than 90% of gastrinomas and non-functioning neuroendocrine tumors [6]. Alterations of the K-*ras* oncogene and the *p53* tumor suppressor gene, both frequently mutated in tumors of the exocrine pancreas, were not identified in NPTs, and therefore are not likely to play an important role in NPT tumorigenesis [7, 8].

Recently, the putative tumor suppressor gene *DPC4* (deleted in pancreatic carcinoma, locus 4) was identified at human chromosome 18q21.1 [9]. DPC4 is a member of the highly conserved family of Smad proteins that are involved in the transduction of signals from the transforming growth factor family of cytokines; *DPC4* has subsequently been designated as *Smad4* [10]. *DPC4* was found to be inactivated, either by homozygous deletion or by point mutation together with a chromosomal deletion, in half of pancreatic carcinomas (9, 11). This finding prompted us to investigate whether *DPC4/Smad4* inactivation plays also a role in the tumorigenesis of NPTs.

2. Material and Methods

2.1 Tumor samples

Twenty-five NPTs (11 insulinomas, 9 non-functioning neuroendocrine carcinomas, 3 gastrinomas, and 2 vipomas) were obtained from the tissue bank of the Department of Surgery, Philipps-Universtiy of Marburg. Tissue specimens included 19 fresh-frozen and 6 paraffin-embedded tumors. All tumor samples used for DNA isolation had a neoplastic cellularity of at least 80% after microdissection of the nonneoplastic tissue. Constitutional normal DNA derived, either from blood lymphocytes or from normal pancreatic tissue, was available from 12 patients.

2.2. PCR and SSCP

PCR amplification was performed with 10 to 20ng of the isolated genomic DNA and 0.5 units *Taq* polymerase (Perkin Elmer, Weiterstadt) in 1.5 or 1.25 or 1.0 mM $MgCl_2$, 10 mM Tris-HCl pH 8.3, 50 mM KCl, 1 mM each primer, 200 mM each dNTP, 5 % dimethyl sulfoxide, and 0.1 mCi of [α^{33}P]dCTP in a final volume of 10 ml. The mixture was subjected to 30-35 cycles of the following program: denaturation at 95 °C for 30 s, primer annealing at 55-58 °C for 30 s, and primer extension at 72 °C for 30 s. The primers for SSCP analysis of exons 8 to 11 that were designed to amplify a fragment length of 250bp or less have previously beendescribed [12]. The PCR products were electrophoresed as described previously [13]. The resulting products were visualized by autoradiography. The presence of abnormally migrating DNA bands was confirmed in several independent PCR reactions loaded on different gels.

2.3. Sequence Analysis

Aberrant bands were cut from the gel, eluted, and reamplified by PCR using the original PCR primers. The resulting products were either directly sequenced by cycle sequencing (SequiTherm, Epicentre) or, in cases where it proved difficult to isolate the aberrant band without contamination from the nearby normal band, the PCR product was first ligated into the pCRII TA-cloning vector (Invitrogen) and then eight to ten independent clones were sequenced (SequiTherm, Epicentre). To distinguish PCR errors from tumor-specific alterations, mutations were only scored when at least half of the clones showed the sequence alteration.

2.4. Loss of Heterozygosity Analysis

Microsatellite markers D18S363, D18S877, D18S474, D18535 and D18S46 from the *DPC4*-region have been used to analyze loss of heterozygosity [11]. PCR amplification and PCR product analysis were performed as described [14]. Loss of heterozygosity (LOH) was defined as a >50% reduction in intensity by visual inspection in either of the two alleles as compared to those in constitutional normal DNA.

3. Results and Discussion

We screened the highly conserved COOH-terminal domain of the *DPC4* gene for mutations in 25 microdissected NPT`s (11 insulinomas, 9 non-functioning neuroendocrine pancreatic carcinomas (NNPC), 3 gastrinomas and 2 vipomas). Exons 8 to 11 were successfully amplified in 24 tumors. Despite repeated attempts, DNA from the NNPC specimen 5955T which had a neoplastic cellularity of 90% failed to give rise to amplification products of *DPC4* exons 8 to 11. In addition, multiplex PCR with primers specific for *DPC4* exon 2 together with primers for K-*ras* exon 1 failed to generate a specific *DPC4* amplification product whereas the specific K-*ras* PCR product was readily detectable . The quality of the tumor DNA was further assured by successful amplification exon 5 and 6 of TP53, resulting in a slightly larger PCR product than expected for the *DPC4* specific amplification. We conclude from these experiments, that homozygous deletion of *DPC4* is a likely explanation for the failure to generate a *DPC4* specific PCR product in this tumor specimen.

SSCP analysis revealed a reproducible abnormal banding pattern in all five control DNA samples derived from pancreatic xenografts which were known to harbor *DPC4* mutations [9]. Upon SSCP analysis of the primary tumor samples using identical conditions reproducibly aberrant bands were seen in 5 of 24 tumors, four of these being NNPCs. Sequence analysis of the aberrant SSCP products identified point mutations or small intragenic deletions of the *DPC4* sequence in all 4 NNPCs (Table 1). In tumor 4176T, the only mutation-positive tumor where constitutional normal DNA from the patient was available, the somatic nature of the mutation could be demonstrated. In addition, LOH of all informative 18q21 markers was seen in this tumor, supporting the concept of biallelic inactivation of the *DPC4* tumor suppressor gene. Of all the other tumor types only the insulinoma 90aT revealed a band shift in exon 8. Sequencing of the variant band revealed a silent base change (TTT to TTC) at codon 362. This alteration was also found in the normal constitutional DNA and the tumor did not show LOH of 18q21 sequences. Therefore this alteration represents most likely a benign polymorphism.

Specimen	Tumor type	TNM	Exon	Codon	Mutation	Effect
90aT	insulinoma	/	8	362	TTT to TTC*	none
19377/94T	NNPT	G2T2N1M1	8	319-330	del 37 bp	frameshift
			8	369	AAT to GAT	Asn to Asp
4176/95T	NNPT	G2T2N0M1	10	457	GCA to TCA	Ala to Ser
818/96T	NNPT	G2T2N1M0	11	515	AGA to TGA	Arg to Stop
MB6T	NNPT	G3 T2N1M1	11	529/530	del TTCA	frameshift
5955/95T	NNPT	G3 T3N1M1	/	/	/	HD

*, polymorphism; HD, homozygous deletion

Table 1: DPC4 alterations in Neuroendocrine Pancreatic Tumors

To our knowledge this is the first report of *DPC4/Smad4* genetic alterations in pancreatic neuroendocrine tumors. Our data suggest that mutational inactivation of the *DPC4* gene is a frequent event in NNPCs, whereas they do not play a significant role in insulinomas, gastrinomas and vipomas. In addition, the one NNPC where we were unable to amplify *DPC4* specific sequences is suggestive for homozygous deletion of the *DPC4* gene region as a second mode of gene inactivation being also operative in this tumor type. Of note, it is likely that the *DPC4* inactivation frequency is underestimated in our study for the following reasons: the mutation analysis was restricted to exons 8 to 11 of *DPC4*, which together span the entire conserved COOH-terminal Smad homology region. However, because 90% of the *DPC4* mutations reported thus far are located in the C-terminal region, the number of undetected mutations is expected to be low [9, 15-25]. The PCR-based detection of homozygous deletions, a mechanism of gene inactivation known to be important for the *DPC4* gene [9, 15, 16], is complicated in primary tumor specimens by the presence of infiltrating nonneoplastic tissue. We attempted to minimize contamination from nonneoplastic tissue by microdissecting the tumor to enrich for the neoplastic cell fraction. Although we achieved by this approach a neoplastic cellularity of at least 80% in all tumor samples, the remaining nonneoplastic cell fraction (up to 20%) is likely to preclude a valid assessment of the homozygous deletion status for some of our cases. SSCP has been shown to be a highly sensitive method to identify mutations in PCR-generated fragments, nevertheless certain mutations may not be detected using this method. Furthermore, it is possible that some of the primary tumors in our collection had large intragenic deletions of *DPC4*, we would have missed, given the strategy for mutation detection used herein. Finally, loss of *DPC4* function due to defects in transcriptional regulation, as shown for example for the *p16* gene, would also have been missed upon analysis of genomic DNA.

To date significant frequencies of mutational *DPC4* inactivation have been found only in a few tumor types such as pancreatic adenocarcinoma xenografts (50%), colorectal carcinoma (17%) and biliary tract cancer (16%), whereas only a minority (<7%) of cancers from other anatomic sides revealed *DPC4* mutations [9, 15-25]. Our finding of *DPC4* alterations in 55% of NNPCs suggest for this tumor type the highest *DPC4* mutation rate reported in any primary tumor so far. The mutational spectrum of *DPC4* in NNPCs seems to be different from those in exocrine pancreatic adenocarcinomas. In pancreatic adenocarcinomas the frequency of inactivation of the *DPC4* gene by point mutations or small intragenic deletions is less compared to the frequencyof homozygous deletions of the *DPC4* region, 20% and 30% respectively [9]. In contrast, forNNPCs point mutations and small deletions appeared to be the predominant inactivation mechanism (4 of 5 tumors). Although more tumors of this type need to be analyzed to firmly establish the mutation frequency in NNPCs, our data clearly support an important role of *DPC4* in the carcinogenesis of NNPC.

It remains speculative why NNPCs are a main target for *DPC4* inactivation and none of the other neuroendocrine pancreatic tumor types. In this regard, it is notable, that all 5 NNPC patients with *DPC4* mutations had an advanced tumor state with lymph node metastases, four of these already having liver metastases at the time of surgery. In contrast, of the four mutation-negative NNPCs none had liver metastases and only one tumor had metastasized into the lymph nodes, while the majority of insulinomas and gastrinomas had a benign phenotype. Therefore, it is tempting to hypothesize that the occurrence of *DPC4* alterations are important for this tumor type to develop a malign phenotype, or even more important to develop a metastatic potential.

Taken together, our data suggest inactivation of *DPC4* is the second most common genetic event besides alterations in the *p16* tumor suppressor gene [6] in NNPCs. Furthermore, the frequency of *DPC4* alteration my rival the frequency found in pancreatic adenocarcinomas and this should stimulate further research using this tumor type as a model system to investigate the tumor suppressivefunction of *DPC4*, helping to refine our picture of the role *DPC4* signaling is playing in tumorigenesis

Literature

[1] A.J. Edis *et al.*, (eds.) Manual of endocrine surgery. Berlin, Heidelberg, New York: Springer-Verlag, (1984).

[2] D. Trump *et al.*,Clinical studies of multiple endocrine neoplasia type 1 (MEN 1). Q. J. Medicine **89** (1996) 653-669.

[3] S.C. Chandrasekharappa *et al.*, Positional cloning of the gene for multiple endocrine neoplasia type 1. Science (Washington DC) **276** (1997) 404-407.

[4] Z. Zhuang Z. *et al.*, Somatic mutations of the MEN1 tumor suppressor gene in sporadic gastrinomas and insulinomas. Cancer Res. **57** (1997) 4682-4686.

[5] B. Evers *et al.*, Gastrinomas demonstrate amplification of the HER-2/neu proto-oncogene. Ann. Surg. **219** (1994) 596-605.

[6] P. Muscarella *et al.*, Genetic alterations in gastrinomas and nonfunctioning neuroendocrine tumors: an analysis of *p16/MTS1* tumor suppressor gene inactivation. Cancer Res. **558** (1998) 237-240.

[7] K. Yoshimoto *et al.*, *Ras* mutations in endocrine tumors: mutation detection by polymerase chain reaction - sigle strand conformation polymorphism. Cancer Res. **83** (1992) 1057-1062.

[8] T. Yashiro *et al.*, Comparison of mutations of ras oncogene in human pancreatic exocrine and endocrine tumors. Surgery **114** (1993) 758-764.

[9] S.A. Hahn *et al.*, *DPC4*, a candidate tumor suppressor gene at human chromosome 18q21.1. Science (Washington DC) **271** (1996) 350-353.

[10] J. Massagué, TGFβ signaling: receptors, transducers, and Mad proteins. Cell **85** (1996) 947-950.

[11] S. A. Hahn *et al.*, Homozygous deletion map at 18q21.1 in pancreatic cancer. Cancer Res. **56** (1996) 490-494.

[12] S.A. Hahn *et al.*, Mutations of the *DPC4/Smad4* gene in biliary tract cancers. Cancer Res. **58** (1995) 1124-1126.

[13] D. Bartsch *et al.*, Cancer **14** (1995) 189-195.

[14] S. A. Hahn *et al.*, Allelotype of pancreatic adenocarcinomas using xenograft enrichment. Cancer Res. **55** (1995) 4670-4675.

[15] M. Schutte *et al., DPC4* gene in various tumor types. Cancer Res. **56** (1996) 2527-2530.

[16] S. Thiagalingam *et al.*, Evaluation of candidate tumor suppressor genes on chromosome 18 in colorectal cancers. Nat. Genet. **13** (1996) 342-346.

[17] Y. Takagi *et al.*, Somatic alterations of the *DPC4* gene in human colorectal cancers in vivo. Gastroenterology **111** (1996) 1369-1372.

[18] M. Nagatake *et al.*, Somatic *in vivo* alterations of the *DPC4* gene at 18q21 in human lung cancers. Cancer Res. **56** (1996) 2718-2720.

[19] A. T. M. Hoque *et al.*, *DPC4* gene mutation in colitis associated neoplasia. Gut **40** (1997) 120-122.

[20] S. K. Kim, *et al.*, *DPC4*, a candidate tumor suppressor gene, is altered infrequently in head and neck squamous cell carcinoma. Cancer Res. **56** (1996) 2519-2521.

[21] M. T. Barrett *et al.*, Allelic loss and mutational analysis of the *DPC4* gene in esophageal adenocarcinoma. Cancer Res. **56** (1996) 4351-4353.

[22] J. Lei *et al.*, Infrequent *DPC4* gene mutation in esophageal cancer, gastric cancer and ulcerative colitis-associated neoplasms. Oncogene **13** (1996) 2459-2462.

[23] X T. Kong *et al.,* Expression and mutational analysis of the *DCC*, *DPC4*, and *MADR2/JV18-1* genes in neuroblastoma. Cancer Res. **57** (1997) 3772-3778.

[24] D. McGrogan *et al.*, Comparative mutational analysis of *DPC4* (Smad4) in prostatic and colorectal carcinomas. Oncogene **15** (1997) 1111-1114.

[25] J. R. Howe *et al.*, Mutations in the *Smad4/DPC4* gene in juvenile polyposis. Science (Washington DC) **280** (1998) 1086-1088.

Molecular Pathogenesis of Pancreatic Cancer
T.M. Gress (Ed.)
IOS Press, 2000

Prevalence of K-*ras* mutations at diagnosis and serum levels of DDT, DDE, PCBs and other organochlorine compounds in exocrine pancreatic cancer

Miquel Porta[1], Manuel Jariod[1], Núria Malats[1], Joan O. Grimalt[2], Alfredo Carrato[3], Luisa Guarner[4], Antonio Salas[5], Juli Rifà[6], Josep M. Corominas[7], Juan Alguacil[1], Montserrat Andreu[7] and Francisco X. Real[1] for the PANKRAS II Study Group

[1] *Institut Municipal d'Investigació Mèdica (IMIM), Universitat Autònoma de Barcelona, Universitat Pompeu Fabra, Carrer del Dr. Aiguader 80, E-08003 Barcelona, Spain;* [2] *Institute of Chemical and Environmental Research (CSIC), Barcelona, Spain;* [3] *Hospital General de Elche, Alicante, Spain;* [4] *Hospital Vall d'Hebron, Barcelona;* [5] *Hospital Mútua de Terrassa, Barcelona, Spain;* [6] *Hospital Son Dureta, Mallorca, Spain;* [7] *Hospital del Mar, Barcelona, Spain*

The possibility that organochlorine compounds play a role in the pathogenesis of exocrine pancreatic cancer through modulation of K-*ras* effects could have significant implications for research on the carcinogenic process of this and other malignancies associated with K-*ras* mutations. Future studies should be based on mechanistic scenarios that integrate evidence from molecular biology, molecular pathology, molecular epidemiology, genetic toxicology, clinical medicine, and environmental chemistry. Whereas organochlorine compounds are ubiquitous throughout the planet and have a wide range of physiologic effects, no clinical or public health inferences are warranted until our findings are replicated in new studies.

1. Introduction

Over 10 years after their high prevalence at diagnosis was first reported, point mutations in the K-*ras* gene remain the most consistent genetic alteration in exocrine pancreatic cancer (EPC). Yet, evidence in support of the hypothesis that the occurrence or the persistence of these mutations may be related to some type of environmental factors has been elusive, perhaps because no empirical data were available for humans. Recently, our group reported that patients with K-*ras* mutated EPC had higher serum concentrations of organochlorine compounds than EPC cases with wild-type K-*ras* [1]. The possibility that organochlorine compounds play a role in the pathogenesis of EPC through modulation of K-*ras* effects could have significant implications for research on the carcinogenic process of this and other malignancies where alterations in *ras* genes are frequent. It could also help to clarify the relationship between organochlorine compounds and the risks of several other neoplasms [1].

Agents such as 1,1,1-trichloro-2,2-bis(p-chlorophenyl)-ethane (p,p'-DDT), its main metabolite and environmental degradation product, 1,1-dichloro-2,2-bis(p-chlorophenyl)-ethylene (p,p'-DDE), several polychlorinated biphenyls (PCBs), hexachlorobenzene and hexachlorocyclohexane comprise the bulk of organochlorine residues in human tissues.

These compounds are ubiquitous throughout the planet, poorly excreted due to their lipophilic properties, and stored in many human tissues [2-9]. DDT was widely used in the past as a pesticide, and it continues to be used, mainly for controlling malaria; total global use (worldwide) may be as great at present as it was in the 1970s [2]. PCBs have been used in insulating and cooling electrical equipment (transformers, capacitators, fluorescent lamps), paints, inks, carbonless copy paper, adhesives, resins, plasticisers and many other products and processes [5-9].

2. Subjects and Methods

A detailed description of methods has been published elsewhere [1,10-13]. Incident cases of EPC were prospectively identified and interviewed during hospital stay. Among 185 patients with EPC, mutations in codon 12 of the K-*ras* gene were determined for 121 using a PCR-RFLP approach [1]; of them 94 (77.7%) harboured mutations, and 27 did not. For the present study, we selected all 17 cases with wild-type K-*ras* tumours from whom at least 3 mL of serum were available. These wild-type cases were frequency matched (1:2 ratio) to cases with a K-*ras* mutated tumour (n=34) for age and sex.

3. Results and Discussion

There were no major differences between the 51 selected cases and the remaining 134 cases with respect to a broad range of personal and lifestyle factors (table 1). Symptom history and characteristics at presentation did not differ significantly either between the two groups (table 2). Thus, our results seem generalisable to a fairly unbiased group of EPC patients.

In studies on organochlorine compounds it is common to find patients whose concentration of a given compound falls below the limit of detection or lies between such limit and the limit of quantitation. However, there is no general agreement among epidemiologists as to how statistical analyses should deal with these values. Figure 1a shows the distribution of values for DDT analogues. Levels of p,p'-DDT were detectable in 36 of the 51 cases (71%); in 6 cases (12%) they were detectable but not quantifiable. All 51 cases of EPC had detectable concentrations of p,p'-DDE, and these were quantifiable in 92% of subjects. Ten PCB congeners were detected; for 7 of them (IUPAC numbers 28, 52, 101, 118, 170, 187 and 194) over half of cases had non-detectable or non-quantifiable levels (figure 2a), and they were thus no longer considered. By contrast, all 51 cases of EPC had detectable levels of congeners 153 and 180, and 43 cases (84%) of PCB 138. The corresponding distribution for the rest of organochlorine compounds is shown in figure 3a. Hexachlorobenzene and β-hexachlorocyclohexane were detected in all cases.

In our study, limits of detection and quantitation were 0.1 and 0.3 ng/mL, respectively (detailed figures for all compounds are available from the authors). When organochlorine serum concentrations were not detected we assigned a value of zero. When a compound was detected but the concentration was under the quantitation threshold, the mid-value between detection and quantitation limits was assigned. The resulting values are shown in table 3, as well as in figures 1b, 2b and 3b (the horizontal line of the box plot represents the median value).

The Total PCBs value was the arithmetic sum of the concentrations of all PCB congeners after value imputation (as described in the previous paragraph). Exposure to PCBs was analysed with a congener-specific approach (i.e., each congener separately), as recommended [8,9]. The variable Total PCBs was used only in multivariate analyses to further adjust DDT and DDE levels (i.e., to separate the effects of DDT and DDE from the effects of PCBs). There were two reasons to do so. First, as mentioned, levels of 7 congeners were often undetected or unquantifiable in the patients (figure 2a, table 3), and the resulting Total PCBs was a construct substantially based on imputed values. Second, Total PCBs mixes congeners with different persistence, hormonal activities, cytochrome P450 inducibility, and carcinogen-promoting potential [1,5-9]. For descriptive purposes, and to enable comparison with other studies, table 3 presents several statistics, both on a wet basis (nanograms per milliliter, which is equivalent to parts per billion [ppb]), and on a lipid basis (expressed as micrograms of the organochlorine compound per gram of Total Lipids). The compound present at highest concentrations was p,p'-DDE, followed by β-hexachlorocyclohexane and hexachlorobenzene (table 3, figures 1b and 3b).

Table 1. Personal and lifestyle characteristics of exocrine pancreatic cancer cases sampled and not sampled for serum organochlorine analyses

Characteristic	Sampled for organochlorine analyses		
	Yes (N= 51)	No (N = 134)	P
Age (years)	65.9±11.9	67.2±12.9	0.561†
Median	67.0	67.7	0.599¶
Gender (% males)	54.9	61.2	0.541§
Education (%) (a)			0.462*
Illiterate	11.8	12.4	
Can only read and write	21.6	29.2	
Up to 10 years of schooling	60.8	47.8	
>10 years of schooling	5.9	10.6	
Occupation (%) (b)			0.511*
Managers, professionals	15.7	17.5	
Service workers	13.7	12.3	
Skilled agricultural & fishery workers	31.4	26.3	
Craft & related trades workers	37.3	21.9	
Plant & machine operators & assemblers	23.5	33.3	
Elementary occupations	45.1	44.7	
Smoking			
Ever-smokers (%)	56.9	55.3	0.983§
Pack-years	23.6±27.7	23.3±32.3	0.949†
Coffee drinking			
Regular coffee drinkers (%)	78.4	88.5	0.147§
No. cups per week	13.3±12.0	12.6±11.6	0.617†
Alcohol drinking			0.517¶
Non-drinker	17.6	13.3	
Occasional drinker	11.8	11.5	
Low consumption	33.3	32.7	
High consumption	15.7	20.4	
Heavy drinker	21.6	22.1	

Plus-minus values are means ± standard deviation (SD). †Student's *t*-test. §Chi-square test. ¶Wilcoxon 2-sample rank sum test. *Fisher's exact test (two-tail). (a) Education data available for all 51 cases and for 113 of the 134 cases (164/185=88.6%). (b) Groups from the International Standard Classification of Occupations (ISCO88). One subject may have had more than one occupation. Occupational data available for 51 cases and 114 of the 134 cases (89.2%).

Table 2. Symptom history and characteristics at presentation of exocrine pancreatic cancer cases sampled and not sampled for organochlorine analyses

Characteristic	Sampled for organochlorine analyses		P *
	Yes (N= 51)	No (N = 134)	
Days from first symptom to diagnosis	112.9±108.3	102.9±118.2	0.599†
Median	82	67	0.150¶
Signs and symptoms (%)			
Weight loss	84.3	84.9	1.000
Asthenia	88.2	85.0	0.644
Anorexia	82.4	82.7	1.000
Vomiting	39.2	31.1	0.300
Nausea	58.8	47.7	0.191
Diarrhea	50.9	40.9	0.247
Steatorrhea	27.5	24.2	0.705
Hypocholia	49.0	56.4	0.410
Choluria	47.1	63.2	0.065
Jaundice	49.0	58.7	0.250
Pruritus	33.3	31.8	0.861
Abdominal pain	66.7	75.2	0.269
Right upper quadrant abdominal pain	53.6	60.6	0.462
Left upper quadrant abdominal pain	56.1	40.7	0.101
Epigastrical pain	80.5	67.6	0.157
Back pain	42.6	51.2	0.391
Physical exam at admission			
Cachexia	11.8	12.9	1.000
Jaundice	45.1	58.3	0.136
Epigastric mass	17.7	5.3	0.016
Right upper quadrant abdominal mass	13.7	15.2	1.000
Left upper quadrant abdominal mass	3.9	3.0	0.671
Courvoisier-Terrier sign	13.7	12.1	0.805
Hepatomegaly	27.5	30.3	0.857
Splenomegaly	7.8	0.8	0.022
Ascites	5.9	4.6	0.711
Stage at diagnosis (%)			0.281§
I	17.6	26.9	
II	17.6	10.4	
II	17.6	10.4	
IV	47.1	50.7	
Missing	0	1.5	
Study interview			
Completed interview (%)	100	84.3	(a)
Duration (minutes)	26.6±7.7	27.2±9.2	0.711†
Median	25.0	25.0	0.565¶

Plus-minus values are means±SD. *Except where otherwise noted, P-values derived from Fisher's exact test. †Student's *t*-test. §Chi-square test. ¶Wilcoxon 2-sample rank sum test. (a) By design: among subjects with available serum, preference was given to those who had been interviewed. Signs and symptoms were elicited from patient interview and clinical records, and disagreements systematically assessed by oncologists on the basis of clinical consistency.

Figure 1a

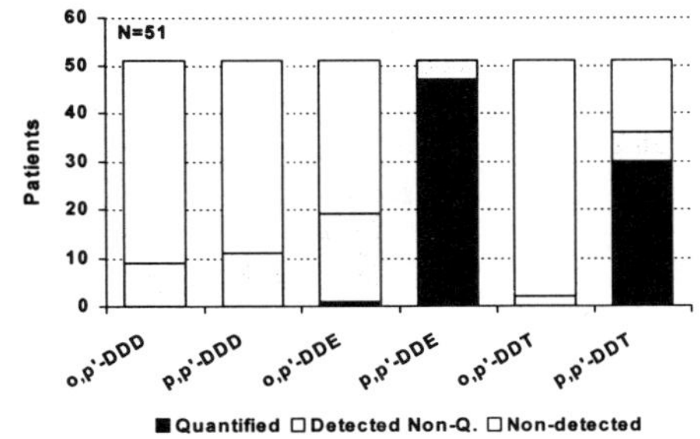

Figure 1b

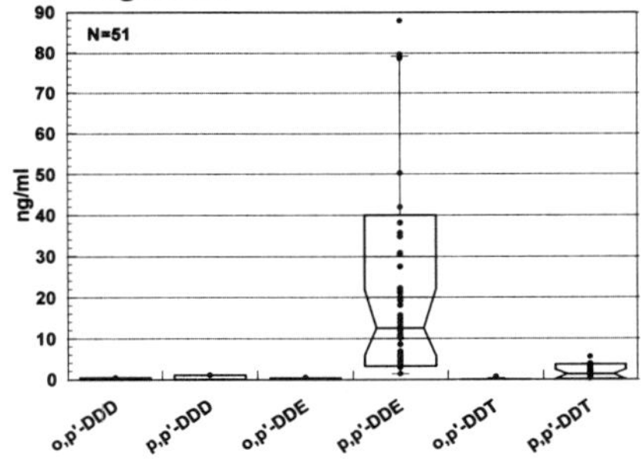

Figure 2a

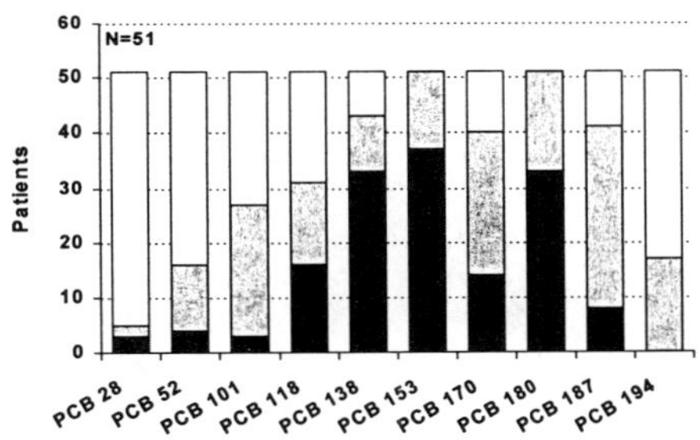

Figure 2b

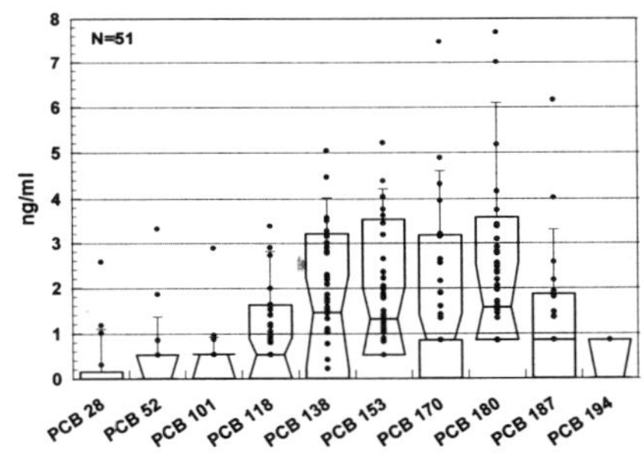

Figure 3a

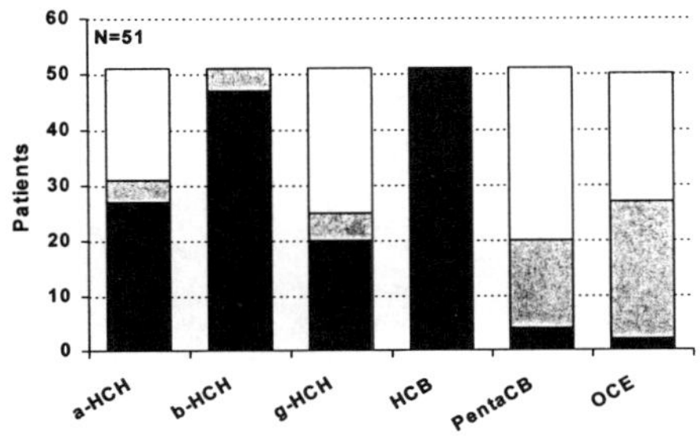

Figure 3b

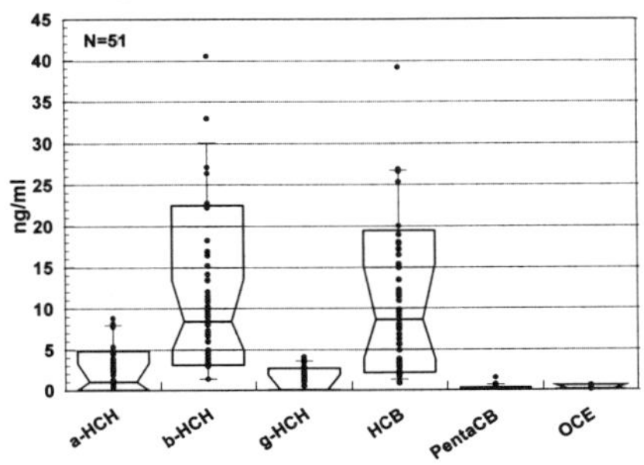

Table 3. PANKRAS II Study: Organochlorine concentrations among cases of exocrine pancreatic cancer (n = 51)

Compound	Percent subjects with levels detected	Percent subjects detected but non-quantified	Wet basis (ng/mL)				Lipid basis (μg/g lipid)			
			Arithmetic mean	SD	Median	Min-Max	Arithmetic mean	SD	Median	Min-Max
p,p'-DDT	70.6	11.8	1.35	1.40	1.20	0.00-5.47	0.21	0.25	0.17	0.00-1.04
p,p'-DDE	100.0	7.8	18.80	19.65	12.49	1.30-87.87	2.73	2.79	1.86	0.14-12.98
p,p'-DDD	21.6	21.6	0.23	0.44	0.00	0.00-1.07	0.04	0.09	0.00	0.00-0.41
o.p'-DDT	3.9	3.9	0.02	0.12	0.00	0.00-0.61	0.01	0.03	0.00	0.00-0.15
o.p'-DDE	37.3	7.8	0.13	0.17	0.00	0.00-0.51	0.02	0.03	0.00	0.00-0.13
o.p'-DDD	17.6	17.6	0.08	0.17	0.00	0.00-0.44	0.01	0.02	0.00	0.00-0.09
PCB 28	9.8	3.9	0.11	0.42	0.00	0.00-2.58	0.02	0.07	0.00	0.00-0.50
PCB 52	31.4	23.5	0.26	0.56	0.00	0.00-3.32	0.04	0.09	0.00	0.00-0.51
PCB 101	52.9	47.1	0.35	0.47	0.54	0.00-2.88	0.05	0.07	0.05	0.00-0.37
PCB 118	60.8	29.4	0.64	0.79	0.53	0.00-3.38	0.09	0.11	0.06	0.00-0.46
PCB 138	84.3	19.6	1.45	1.29	1.45	0.00-5.04	0.21	0.22	0.16	0.00-1.21
PCB 153	100.0	27.5	1.59	1.14	1.31	0.52-5.21	0.24	0.18	0.18	0.05-0.75
PCB 170	78.4	51.0	1.26	1.43	0.85	0.00-7.47	0.20	0.29	0.14	0.00-1.80
PCB 180	100.0	35.3	2.01	1.49	1.56	0.83-7.69	0.30	0.21	0.22	0.10-0.92
PCB 187	80.4	64.7	0.97	1.02	0.85	0.00-6.15	0.14	0.17	0.12	0.00-1.13
PCB 194	33.3	33.3	0.28	0.40	0.00	0.00-0.85	0.05	0.08	0.00	0.00-0.33
"Total PCBs"	—	—	8.91	4.90	7.97	1.58-25.00	1.33	0.76	1.10	0.21-3.66
Hexachlorobenzene	100.0	0.0	10.51	7.86	8.64	0.79-39.13	1.61	1.39	1.08	0.08-6.46
α-hexachlorocyclohexane	60.8	7.8	1.84	2.30	1.01	0.00-8.84	0.29	0.42	0.11	0.00-1.97
β-hexachlorocyclohexane	100.0	7.8	10.67	8.14	8.42	1.35-40.48	1.65	1.40	1.18	0.19-6.46
γ-hexachlorocyclohexane	49.0	9.8	0.90	1.17	0.00	0.00-4.07	0.14	0.20	0.00	0.00-0.65
Octachlorostyrene	54.0	50.0	0.28	0.28	0.31	0.00-0.55	0.04	0.05	0.02	0.00-0.21
Pentachlorobenzene	39.2	31.4	0.14	0.25	0.00	0.00-1.49	0.02	0.04	0.00	0.00-0.26

Serum levels of p,p'-DDT and p,p'-DDE were significantly higher among the 51 cases of EPC than among the 26 hospital controls (table 4). The 51 cases were over 5 times more likely to be in the upper tertile of p,p'-DDE than the 26 controls (multivariate-adjusted odds ratio: 5.6 [95% CI 1.3 - 24.6], p for trend 0.025). The differences were entirely due to the higher levels of cases with mutated tumours, concentrations among cases with wild-type tumours being scarcely different from controls (table 5). The 34 cases with mutated tumours were over 10 times more likely to be in the upper tertile of p,p'-DDE than the 26 controls (multivariate-adjusted odds ratio: 10.5 [95% CI 1.9 - 59.3] (p for trend 0.007). None of the odds ratios comparing wild-type cases and controls was significantly increased.

Table 4. Case-control comparison. Serum concentration among all 51 cases of exocrine pancreatic cancer are compared to concentrations among the 26 hospital controls

Compound	Tertiles (μg / g lipid)	**Crude** OR	**Crude** P for trend (OR 95%CI)	**Adjusted *** OR	**Adjusted *** P for trend (OR 95%CI)
p,p'-DDT	Nd+DNq	1.00	0.040	1.00	0.002
	≤ 0.225	1.41	(0.46-4.36)	2.99	(0.69-12.89)
	> 0.225	4.32	(1.08-17.31)	15.77	(2.68-92.89)
p,p'-DDE	≤ 0.950	1.00	0.052	1.00	0.025
	≤ 2.350	1.00	(0.33-3.01)	1.19	(0.34-4.09)
	> 2.350	3.85	(1.03-14.44)	5.56	(1.26-24.61)

Tertiles based on distribution among 77 patients. Odds ratios (ORs) derived from values individually-adjusted by total lipids. *Adjusted by age, gender, and tobacco, coffee and alcohol consumption. Nd: Non detected. DNq: Detected, non quantifiable.

Table 5. Serum concentrations (median, ng/mL) of p,p'-DDT, p,p'-DDE and the three predominant PCBs among controls, and among cases of exocrine pancreatic cancer with and without mutations in the K-*ras* gene

Compound	**Controls** (n=26)	**Cases of EPC** — **Mutated** (n=34)	**Cases of EPC** — **Wild-type** (n=17)
p,p'-DDT	0.2	1.4 (0.001)	0.2 (0.13)
p,p'-DDE	7.6	14.8 (0.002)	6.8 (0.29)
PCB 138	1.1	1.7 (0.058)	0.2 (0.72)
PCB 153	1.3	1.5 (0.030)	0.8 (0.37)
PCB 180	0.9	2.0 (0.003)	0.9 (0.50)

Values in brackets are the statistical significance (P-value) for differences between controls and mutated cases, and between controls and wild-type cases (covariance analysis, adjusting by total lipids, age, sex, and tobacco, alcohol and coffee consumption).

Acknowledgements

This study was supported in part by research grants from Fondo de Investigación Sanitaria (92/0007, 95/0017 and 97/1138), Fundación Salud 2000, MSD Spain and Generalitat de Catalunya (CIRIT 1995 / SGR 434, CIRIT 1995 / SGR 435 and 1998 / BEAi 400011). The authors are also indebted to R. Otero, A. Serrat, V. Barberà, M. Torà, S. Costafreda, L. Ruiz, M. Soler, D.J. MacFarlane, J. Gomez, P. Barbas and L. Español. Valuable scientific advise was provided by A.J. McMichael, P.G. Toniolo, J. Vila, M. Hernán, A.M. García, K.B. Moysich, M. Kogevinas, H. Vainio, C. Malaveille, M. Luotamo, E.F. Schisterman, D.J. Hunter, F. Laden, I. De Vivo, M.I. Covas, J. Marrugat, F.G. Benavides and J. Sunyer. Partial results of this study were presented at the 16th. Scientific Meeting of the Spanish Society of Epidemiology (Sevilla, 20 - 23 October 1998) (Rev Esp Salud Pública 1998; 72 Supl: 97), at the Second International Congress "Biliopancreatic malignancy: from gene to cure" (Amsterdam, 4 - 6 February 1999), at the Channing Laboratory (Boston, 9 March 1999), at the National Cancer Institute (Rockville, 21 April 1999), and at The University of North Carolina School of Public Health (Chapel Hill, 7 May 1999).

References

[1] M. Porta *et al*, Serum concentrations of organochlorine compounds and K-*ras* mutations in exocrine pancreatic cancer. *The Lancet* 1999; **354**: 2125-2129.

[2] F.Laden *et al*, Environmental risk factors and female breast cancer. *Annual Review of Public Health* 1998; **19**: 101-123.

[3] N.Malats *et al*, DDT and pancreatic cancer. J Natl Cancer Inst 1993; 85: 328.

[4] D.Smith. Worldwide trends in DDT levels in human breast milk *International Journal of Epidemiology* 1999; **28**: 179-188.

[5] United Nation Environment Programme, International Labour Organisation, World Health Organisation. *Polychlorinated dibenzo-para-dioxins and dibenzofurans.* International Programme on Chemical Safety, IPCS. Geneva: World Health Organization, 1989.

[6] J.D. McKinney and C.L.Waller CL, Polychlorinated biphenyls as hormonally active structural analogues. *Environmental Health Perspectives* 1994; **102**: 290-297.

[7] D. Warshawsky, Polycyclic aromatic hydrocarbons in carcinogenesis. *Environmental Health Perspectives* 1999; **107**: 317-319.

[8] K.B. Moysich KB *et al*, An evaluation of proposed frameworks for grouping polychlorinated biphenyl (PCB) congener data into meaningful analytic units. *American Journal of Industrial Medicine* 1999; **35**: 223-231.

[9] M.S. Wolff *et al*, Proposed PCB congener groupings for epidemiological studies. *Environmental Health Perspectives* 1997; **105**: 13-14.

[10] M.Porta *et al*, Association between coffee drinking and K-*ras* mutations in exocrine pancreatic cancer. *Journal of Epidemiology & Community Health* 1999; **53**: 702-709.

[11] M.Soler *et al*, Medical conditions in patients with pancreatic and biliary diseases: Validity and agreement between data from questionnaires and medical records. *Digestive Diseases & Sciences* 1999; **44**: 2469-2477.

[12] M. Porta *et al*, *Estudio multicéntrico prospectivo sobre el papel del oncogen K-ras y del gen p53 en el diagnóstico, el pronóstico y la etiología del cáncer de páncreas exocrino y el cáncer de las vías biliares (PANKRAS II).* Fondo de Investigación Sanitaria, Proyecto #92/0007. Madrid: Fondo de Investigación Sanitaria, Ministry of Health, 1991.

[13] M.Porta *et al*, Role of mutations in K-ras and p53 genes in exocrine pancreatic cancer and cancer of the biliary tract (PANKRAS II). In: Sankaranarayanan R, Wahrendorf J, Démaret E, eds. *Directory of on-going research in cancer epidemiology 1996.* IARC Scientific publications, n°137. Lyon: International Agency for Research on Cancer, 1996: 304.

Molecular Pathogenesis of Pancreatic Cancer
T.M. Gress (Ed.)
IOS Press, 2000

Establishment of a cryopreserved tissue bank and a xenografting facility for pancreatic cancer

C. Sorio, A. Bonora, S. Orlandini, P.S. Moore, P. Capelli, G. Zamboni, P. Cristofori, G. Dal Negro, P. Marchiori, G. Gaviraghi, M. Falconi, P. Pederzoli, A. Scarpa
Dipartimento di Patologia (C.S., S.O., P.S.M., P.C., G.Z., A.S.) e Dipartimento di Chirurgia (A.B., M.F., P.P.), Università di Verona, Italy. GlaxoWellcome S.p.A., Medicines Research Centre, (P.C., G.D.N., P.M., G.G.), Verona, Italy.

Abstract

We assessed the suitability of cryopreserved neoplastic tissues for xenografting into nude mice by comparing the take rate in 21 samples of pancreatic cancer. Twelve fresh samples were directly implanted in *nu/nu* mice while nine were frozen in cryopreserving solution and implanted at a later time. A total of 11 tumors grew in the animals, six from the freshly implanted samples and five from those cryopreserved. Our results demonstrate that the take rate for xenografting is comparable between cryopreserved and fresh tissue samples, and thus it is possible to create a neoplastic tissue bank whose cellular component can be vitally cryopreseved. The procedure allows for the exchange of tumor material between institutions and permits the establishment of centralized facilities for the storage of an array of different primary tumor samples suitable for the production of *in vivo* models of cancers.

INTRODUCTION

The identification of genetic and biochemical alterations in pancreatic cancer has the potential to provide new tools to assess prognosis and find novel therapeutic targets. The availability of cellular models is fundamental for these goals, as the major problem when dealing with ductal carcinoma of the pancreas is the paucity of the neoplastic cells, often embedded within a strong desmoplastic reaction. Sophisticated enrichment techniques, including cryostat enrichment and microscope-driven dissection, have been used to obtain a suitable cancer cellularity from primary cancers for genetic studies [1, 2].

Xenografting human pancreatic cancer in nu/nu mice provides an excellent alternative for several reasons. The success of the implant is much higher compared to the establishment of cell lines from primary tumors [3], thus allowing the establishment of a wider library of neoplastic phenotypes, growing in conditions that more closely resemble the original one. In addition, once established, xenografted tumors may be propagated by implantion into additional mice, showing a high degree of genetic stability during subsequent passages [4] and have been utilized for preclinical studies on drug effects [5, 6]. Finally, the ability of neoplastic clones to establish local or distant metastases associated with specific genetic alterations [4] in nude mice allows the recognition and isolation of selected subclones that would be impossible to recognize *in vitro*.

However, the organization, cost and facilities necessary to obtain such material are beyond the reach of many laboratories due to the complex organization required.

Vital cryopreservation of tumor tissue would allow to overcome some of the issues involved in xenografting. In order to address the possibility of using cryopreserved tissues, we compared the take rate of fresh and cryopreserved material in a newly established pancreatic cancer tissue bank.

METHODS

Two-four week old *nu/nu* Swiss mice were used. The animal research complied with the GlaxoWellcome company policy on the Care and Use of Animals. Fresh surgical specimens of 21 human pancreatic ductal carcinoma were used. Samples were reduced to 1-2 mm^3 fragments and frozen at 1°/min in 10% DMSO, 30% FBS and 60% RPMI 1640 and then transferred to liquid nitrogen. Twelve fresh tissues and nine vitally frozen samples were soaked in Matrigel® and transferred to the animal facility located at Glaxo-Wellcome laboratories. A minimum of three mice were implanted subcutaneously with 2-5 tissue fragments. Tumor formation was checked weekly by visual inspection and palpation. Mice were sacrificed when the tumor reached at least 1 cm in diameter. The tumor was removed and divided in three fragments. The first was frozen and stored at –80 °C, the second reduced in small fragments and cryopreserved in liquid nitrogen and the remaining fixed in formalin for histological analysis. Each neoplasm was subsequently re-implanted in new sets of mice for two to five passages.

RESULTS

Table 1 summarizes the results. The overall success rate was 52% (11/21). Five of the nine (56%) implants of cryopreserved tissue and six of 12 (50%) of fresh tissue fragments led to tumor growth.

CONCLUSIONS

Our results demonstrate that: i) it is possible to cryopreserve human pancreatic tumor fragments without enzymatic dissociation and obtain successful implantation in nu/nu mice; ii) there is no difference in the success rate of growth in *nu/nu* mice between vitally frozen or fresh tissue implants.

Cryopreservation of tissues is used routinely for transplant purposes, while it has not been reported its use to create a vital bank of cancer tissues. Successful tumor take in nude mice has been reported at a frequency ranging from 50% to 80% using fresh primary pancreatic cancer tissues [4, 7, 8]. No information is available comparing the rate of tumor take between fresh and frozen tissue.

Case	Tumor location	Differentiation	Sample	Mice implanted	Mice with tumor growth
PDX1	Head-body	Moderate	Fresh	5	2
PDX2	Head	Moderate	Fresh	5	4
PDX3	Head	Poor	Fresh	5	2
PDX4	Head	Moderate	Fresh	3	2
PDX5	Head	Moderate	Fresh	4	4
PDX6	Head	Poor	Fresh	5	2
PDX7	Head	Poor	Cryopreserved	4	2
PDX8	Head	Poor	Cryopreserved	4	2
PDX9	Head	Moderate	Cryopreserved	3	2
PDX10	Head	Moderate	Cryopreserved	3	1
PDX11	Body-tail	Moderate	Cryopreserved	5	2
DC1	Head	Poor	Fresh	5	none
DC2	Body	Moderate	Fresh	3	none
DC3	Head	Moderate	Fresh	3	none
DC4	Head	Moderate	Fresh	3	none
DC5	Head	Poor	Fresh	3	none
DC6	Head	Moderate	Fresh	4	none
DC7	Head	Poor	Cryopreserved	3	none
DC8	Head	Poor	Cryopreserved	5	none
DC9	Body-tail	Well	Cryopreserved	3	none
DC10	Head	Moderate	Cryopreserved	2	none

Table 1. Pancreatic ductal carcinomas implanted in nu/nu mice.

As we were interested both in establishing a pancreatic ductal carcinoma tissue bank growing in nude mice and in reducing the extent of coordination necessary to implant fresh samples, we processed fresh neoplastic fragments and compared the yield of these implants with those obtained using cryopreserved tissue. We obtained comparable success rates using vitally frozen or fresh tissue implants.

The availability of vitally frozen primary samples offers the advantage to schedule implants in nude mice according to the availability of animals and/or operators, thus allowing relevant time and cost savings. Cryopreserved tissues can also be prepared and stored in any center and delivered at a later time to a xenografting facility. Once the first tumor growth has been obtained, cryopreservation provides a safety reservoir in case of failure of reimplants or mouse death. Furthermore, a frozen bank of vital xenografts allows the storage of a representative series of different cancer geno-phenotypes that can be expanded whenever necessary, thus overcoming the problem of shortage of biological material or the necessity to increase the propagation-related costs and efforts prohibitively.

The use of tissue vital cryopreservation would also allow collection of cancer samples from centers that do not have a nude mice facility and wish to contribute with biological material that can be shipped at a later time. A cryopreserved tissue bank of xenografted pancreatic cancers, once genetically characterized will allow the selection of the most appropriate array of models for experimental applications on drug sensitivity in relation to the genetic and expression profiles.

Acknowledgement

Supported by grants from the Consorzio Studi Universitari di Verona to A.S., Verona, Italy; Associazione Italiana Ricerca Cancro (AIRC) to A.S., Milan, Italy; cofinanced grant from Verona University and Ministero Università e Ricerca Scientifica e Tecnologica to A.S. and G.Z. (MURST, COFIN 9806151968 and 9906195987), Rome, Italy; and European Community grant BIOMED 2 CE-Contract No. BMH4-CT98-3805.

Literature

[1] A. Achille *et al*, Chromosome 7q allelic losses in pancreatic carcinoma. Cancer Res **56** (1996), 3808-3813.

[2] C. Sorio *et al*, The FHIT gene is expressed in pancreatic ductular cells and is altered in pancreatic cancers. Cancer Res **59** (1999), 1308-1314.

[3] X. Fu *et al*, A metastatic nude-mouse model of human pancreatic cancer constructed orthotopically with histologically intact patient specimens. Proc Natl Acad Sci USA **89** (1992), 5645-5649.

[4] G. Reyes *et al*, Orthotopic xenografts of human pancreatic carcinomas acquire genetic aberrations during dissemination in nude mice. Cancer Res **56** (1996), 5713-5719.

[5] R.M. Mohammad *et al*, An orthotopic model of human pancreatic cancer in severe combined immunodeficient mice: potential application for preclinical studies. Clin Cancer Res **4** (1998), 887-894.

[6] F. Bunz *et al*, Disruption of p53 in human cancer cells alters the responses to therapeutic agents. J Clin Invest **104** (1999), 263-269.

[7] J. Bocsi & A. Zalatnai, Establishment and long-term xenografting of human pancreatic carcinomas in immunosuppressed mice: changes and stability in morphology, DNA ploidy and proliferation activity. J Cancer Res Clin Oncol **125** (1999), 9-19.

[8] S.A. Hahn *et al*, Allelotype of pancreatic adenocarcinoma using xenograft enrichment. Cancer Res **55** (1995), 4670-4675.

Molecular pathways implicated in pancreatic ductal cancer are not involved in exocrine nonductal or endocrine pancreatic tumorigenesis

Patrick S. Moore, Gildas Rigaud, Giuseppe Zamboni and Aldo Scarpa
Pathology Department, Section of Anatomical Pathology, Università di Verona, Italy

Pancreatic ductal carcinoma is characterized by a relatively unique molecular fingerprint constituted by activating point mutations at codon 12 of the K-*ras* oncogene in 80% of the cases and inactivation of the tumor suppressor genes *p16*$^{INK4a/}$ (*CDKN2/MTS1*) and *p53* in 90% and 60% of cases, respectively [1, 7, 12, 18, 21, 22, 26]. More recently, the *DPC4/Smad4* gene, a component of the TGF–β signaling pathway, has also been implicated in about half of these cancers [8]. While inactivation of the *p53* gene is usually due to mutation of one allele and the loss of the other [18, 21], such a mechanism is responsible for only a small proportion of *p16* and *DPC4* alterations and in fact, homozygous deletion accounts for up to one-half of alterations of these two genes [6, 8]. The *p16* gene may also be silenced by promoter methylation in a proportion of cases [23].

Very little is known about the molecular abnormalities in pancreatic neoplasms other than ductal, which comprises those tumor entities arising from both the exocrine and endocrine pancreas. We have analyzed 112 primary pancreatic tumors of different types for alterations in the K-*ras*, *p16*, *p53* and *DPC4* genes. In particular, 34 ductal cancers, 37 exocrine nonductal and 41 endocrine tumors have been examined for alterations in the above genes and for allelic loss on chromosomes 9p, 17p, and 18q. We also report the status of these four genes in 27 pancreatic ductal cancer cell lines.

Ductal cancer cell lines. The results of the analysis of the 27 cell lines are summarized in Table 1. Mutations of the K-*ras* and *p53* genes were found in 21 (78%) and 22 (81%) cell lines, respectively. Alterations in the *p16* gene were found in 24 cell lines (89%), consisting in nine homozygous deletions (33%), eight mutations or small deletions (30%) and seven with methylation of the 5' CpG island (26%). Homozygous deletion of the *DPC4* gene was observed in seven cell-lines (26%), while only one mutation was found (4%). Thus, 30% of cases had alteration of *DPC4*. Taken together, 19 of the 27 cell-lines (70%) had concurrent alterations in K-*ras*, *p53*, and *p16*. All eight cell-lines showing abnormalities in *DPC4* had concurrent alteration of all the other three genes analyzed. Only two cell-lines, QGP-1 and SW979, had no detectable alterations in any of these four genes. Our analysis demonstrated that the frequency and pattern of the anomalies in K-*ras*, *p16*, *p53* and *DPC4* in this panel of cell-lines are comparable to those seen in xenografted and primary ductal cancers [2, 11, 19, 24, 26, 28].

Primary ductal carcinomas. In our series of 34 primary ductal adenocarcinomas we found somatic alterations in all four of the genes analyzed at a frequency comparable to or only slightly lower than that observed in our panel of cell lines and in reported xenografted cancers [19]. All mutations were somatic in nature with the exception of the *p16* gene alteration in case PC16, which was germline in origin. Mutations in *DPC4* were found in 9% of cases. Two previously unreported polymorphisms in the *DPC4* gene were found by our SSCP analysis, namely a T-C base change at codon 362 and a C-T substitution at nucleotide 1798 in the 3' untranslated region (Table 2). Based upon previous reports, mutations in *DPC4* would be expected to be somewhat more frequent than found in this panel of cancers [19]. To rule out the possibility that we were not able to detect sequence variants with the PCR fragments used for SSCP, each exon was subsequently analyzed using two fragments less than 180 bp in length. No additional mutations were found, although we were able to detect all *DPC4* mutations by our PCR-SSCP conditions in six xenografted ductal cancers controls. Allelic loss on chromosomes 9p, 17p, and 18q was found in 67%, 65%, and 70% of cases, respectively (Table 2). Given the fact that deletions on chromosome 18q are usually very large and may involve the entire chromosome [9], it is reasonable to suppose that there may be mutational targets in addition to *DPC4*. Taken together, the results of the analysis of our primary ductal cancers are largely concordant with the data derived from both cell-lines and xenografts, giving additional support for the involvement of these genes in the pathogenesis of this malignancy.

Table 1. *Molecular Alterations in Pancreatic Ductal Cancer Cell-Lines*

	K-ras	**p53**	**p16**	**DPC4**
AsPc1	12 GGT-GAT	135 TGC-GC	77 ACT-A	none
A818.4	12 GGT-CGT	none	HD	none
BJ	12 GGT-GAT	275 TGT-TAT	44 TAC-TAAC	HD
CFPAC1	12 GGT-GTT	242 TGC-CGC	methylated	HD
Ger	12 GGT-GAT	272 GTG-TTG	HD	HD
IMIM-PC2	12 GGT-GAT	306 CGA-TGA	HD	none
FG-2	12 GGT-GAT	none	52 ATG-AAG	none
PCJ1	12 GGT-GTT	175 CGC-CAC	HD	355 GAC-GGC
PSK1	12 GGT-CGT	132 AAG-CAG	HD	HD
PT45	none	280 AGA-AAA	HD	none
T3M4	none	220 TAT-TGT	methylated	none
BI	12 GGT-GAT	197 GTG-TTG	methylated	HD
HPAF	12 GGT-GAT	151 CCC-TCC	29-34 del	none
MiaPaCa2	12 GGT-TGT	248 CGG-TGG	HD	none
PaCa3	none	none	methylated	none
PaCa44	12 GGT-GTT	176 TGC-AGC	methylated	none
PANC1	12 GGT-GAT	273 CGT-CAT	HD	none
PANC2	12 GGT-GTT	176 TGC-AGC	methylated	none
SK-PC 1	12 GGT-GAT	282 CGG-CTG	HD	HD
FA6	12 GGT-GAT	149, 840 bp del	58 CGA-TGA	HD
MDAPanc3	12 GGT-GCT	273 CGT-TGT	-36 to (+5)-C	none
PaTu-I	12 GGT-GTT	176 TGC-AGC	methylated	none
QGP-1	none	none	none	none
RWP1	12 GGT-GAT	175 CGC-CAC	58 CGA-TGA	none
Suit-2	12 GGT-GAT	273 CGT-CAT	69 GAG-TAG	none
SW979	none	none	none	none
SW850	none	215 AGT-ATT	none	none
	21/27	***22/27***	***24/27***	***8/27***
	78%	***81%***	***89%***	***30%***

Table 2. *Molecular Alterations in Primary Pancreatic Ductal Cancers*

	K-ras	p53	p16	DPC4
PC3	12 GGT-GAT	157-158, 5 bp del	none	none
PC4	12 GGT-GAT	none	90 TTC-TTTC	none
PC5	none	249 AGG-ATG	none	none
PC6	none	266 GGA-TGA	none	none
PC9	none	40 AGT-GT	none	none
PC11	12 GGT-AGT	none	44 TAC-TAAC	441, 58bp-TG
PC13	12 GGT-GTT	none	none	nt 1798 C-T
PC14	12 GGT-GTT	219 CCC-CC	none	none
PC15	12 GGT-GAT	none	none	none
PC16	12 GGT-GTT	249 AGG-AGT	48 CCG-ACG	none
PC17	12 GGT-GTT	none	methylated	none
PC18	12 GGT-GTT	273 CGT-TGT	none	nt 1798 C-T
PC19	12 GGT-GTT	132 AAG-AGG	none	none
PC20	12 GGT-GAT	152 CCG-G	none	none
PC21	12 GGT-GAT	249 AGG-GGG	none	none
PC22	12 GGT-GTT	none	methylated	none
PC23	12 GGT-GAT	none	none	362 TTT-TTC
PC24	none	none	148 GCG-ACG	none
PC25	12 GGT-GTT	243, 7 bp ins	none	none
PC26	12 GGT-GTT	none	methylated	none
PC27	12 GGT-GAT	none	none	523 TGC-TGG
PC28	12 GGT-GAT	none	none	none
PC29	12 GGT-GAT	177 CCC-CGC	57-59 del	none
PC30	12 GGT-GAT	none	77 ACT-A	none
PC31	none	none	110 TGG-TAG	none
PC32	none	none	none	493 GAT-AAT
PC33	12 GGT-GTT	248 CGG-CAG	94 CTG-CGG	none
PC34	12 GGT-GTT	273 CGT-CAT	none	none
PC35	12 GGT-CGT	273 CGT-CTT	methylated	none
PC36	12 GGT-CGT	282 CGG-TGG	55, 10 bp ins	none
PC37	12 GGT-GAT	none	none	none
PC38	12 GGT-GAT	214 CAT-CGT	148 GCG-ACG	none
PC39	12 GGT-GTT	175 CGC-CAC	none	none
	28/34	***18/34***	***13/24***	***3/34***
	82%	***53%***	***38%***	***9%***

Intraductal papillary mucinous tumors. To date, only K-*ras* mutations have been found in IPMT at varying frequency [14, 20, 25, 29]. *p53* mutations are rare and associated with the invasive component of the tumor [25]. In ten cryostat-enriched cases of IPMT, seven of which had an invasive cancer component, we found three K-*ras* mutations and no alteration of either *p16*, *p53* or *DPC4*. It would seem reasonable to consider IPMT a tumor entity with molecular targets involved in its pathogenesis distinct from those of ductal carcinoma. The low frequency of LOH found on chromosomes 9p, 17p, and 18q further substantiates this supposition.

Acinar cancers. In acinar cell carcinoma, mutations in K-*ras* are exceedingly rare [10, 27] and *p53* mutation has not been found in the three cases previously analyzed [17]. Our six acinar carcinomas showed no K-*ras* mutations and frequent allelic losses on chromosomes 9p, 17p and 18q. However, our mutational analysis showed that the targets of these chromosomal losses are not *p16*, *p53*, or *DPC4*.

Solid pseudopapillary tumors. Neither *ras* gene family mutations nor alterations in *p53* have been found in solid-papillary tumors [3, 16]. Our five cases confirmed this data. We found no alterations in either *p16* or *DPC4* and no allelic losses on either 9p, 17p or 18q were detected. Thus, the molecular events leading to this peculiar entity remain elusive.

Table 3. *Molecular Alterations in Primary Pancreatic Ampullary Cancers*

	K-ras	p53	p16	DPC4
AT1	none	245 GGC-GAC	none	none
AT3	none	220 TAT-TGT	methylated	none
AT4	12 GGT-GAT	none	none	none
AT5	none	245 GGC-CGC	methylated	none
AT6	none	179 CAT-TAT	none	none
AT7	none	none	none	none
AT8	none	219 CCC-CC	none	none
AT9	12 GGT-GCT	173 GTG-ATG	none	none
AT12	none	282 CGG-CTG	none	none
AT13	12 GGT-GAT	213 CGA-TGA	148 GCG-ACG	none
AT14	12 GGT-GAT	none	methylated	none
AT15	none	none	148 GCG-ACG	none
AT17	12 GGT-GAT	none	none	none
AT19	12 GGT-GAT	175 CGC-CAC	none	350-355 del
AT60	not done	not done	none	none
AT61	12 GGT-GCT	none	methylated	none
	7/16	***9/16***	***4/16***	***1/16***
	44%	***56%***	***25%***	***6%***

Ampulla of Vater Tumors. In our series of 16 cancers composed of small neoplasms of unequivocal ampullary origin, alterations were found in all four genes, with *p53* mutations being the most frequent event (56%), accompanied in the majority of cases by the loss of the second allele. K-*ras* mutations were detected in 44% of cases. One case had a mutation in the *DPC4* gene (6%), while four cases had inactivation of *p16* (25%), all of which were represented by *de novo* methylation. The most frequent allelic losses were on chromosome 17p (63%). Multigenic analysis showed that 75% (12/16) of ampullary cancers had alterations in two of the K-*ras*, *p53* or *p16* genes, with no apparent preference for any particular combination. Allelic loss on chromosomes 9p, 17p, and 18q was detected in 13%, 56% and 50% of cases (Table 3). Allelic loss on chromosome 18q was a relatively frequent event (50%), while chromosome 9p LOH was infrequent (13%). Thus ampullary cancers have molecular alterations in the same genes implicated in ductal cancers. Although the frequencies of alterations are somewhat different, this would imply that similar molecular pathways are involved in ductal and ampullary cancers.

Endocrine tumors. The series of 41 pancreatic endocrine tumors was composed of 30 nonfunctioning and 11 functioning tumors, including nine insulinomas, 1 gastrinoma and 1 VIPoma. One nonfunctioning case had a mutation in K-*ras,* another nonfunctioning tumor had a mutated *p53* gene and one insulinoma was found to harbor a *p16* mutation affecting a splice junction. Our data confirm the extreme rarity of mutations in either K-*ras* or *p53* in these tumors [4, 15]. No alterations were found in *DPC4*. LOH on chromosome 17p was found in 54% of nonfunctional cases, but in only 8% of functioning cancers. This supports a previous suggestion indicating the presence of a tumor suppressor gene other than *p53* on chromosomal arm 17p, which is involved in nonfunctional PET tumorigenesis [4]. Chromosome 9p allelic loss was seen in a low proportion in both nonfunctional (22%) and functional tumors (20%) and would suggest that alteration of this gene is not of paramount importance in endocrine tumorigenesis. No case showed alteration in the *DPC4* gene, in spite of the finding of a moderately frequent LOH on chromosome 18q, including 29% of nonfunctional and 38% of functional tumors.

Conclusions. The frequency and combination of mutations in these four genes in primary ductal cancers is similar to that seen in our panel of 27 ductal cancer cell lines and comparable to that described in xenografted cancers. Of importance, the comprehensive data regarding the multigenic alterations present in this large series of cell-lines may prove valuable for studies involving drug sensitivity or resistance that may be associated with inactivation of a particular gene or molecular pathway [5, 13]. Only carcinomas arising from the epithelium of pancreatic ducts and their terminal excretory structure (ampulla of Vater) have common molecular features. The genetic pathways implicated in ductal cancer are not involved in the pathogenesis of exocrine nonductal and endocrine tumors. These neoplasms must therefore have distinct molecular pathways involved in tumorigenesis. This likelihood seems highly plausible when considered together with the fact that each tumor type has a distinct pathological and clinical features, including dramatic differences in patient survival.

This study was supported by grants from the Associazione Italiana Ricerca Cancro (AIRC), Milan, Italy; Consorzio Studi Universitari di Verona, Italy; cofinanced grant (COFIN98-COFIN99) from Verona University and Ministero Università e Ricerca Scientifica e Tecnologica (MURST), Rome, Italy; and BIOMED 2 CE-Contract No. BMH4-CT98-3805.

Literature

[1] C. Almoguera, *et al.*, Most human carcinomas of the exocrine pancreas contain mutant c-K-ras genes. Cell **53** (1988), 549-554.

[2] C.M. Barton, *et al.*, Abnormalities of the p53 tumour suppressor gene in human pancreatic cancer. Br J Cancer **64** (1991), 1076-1082.

[3] D. Bartsch, *et al.*, K-ras oncogene mutations indicate malignancy in cystic tumors of the pancreas. Ann Surg **228** (1998), 79-86.

[4] S. Beghelli, *et al.*, Pancreatic endocrine tumours: evidence for a tumour suppressor pathogenesis and for a tumour suppressor gene on chromosome 17p. J Pathol **186** (1998), 41-50.

[5] F. Bunz, *et al.*, Disruption of p53 in human cancer cells alters the responses to therapeutic agents. J Clin Invest **104** (1999), 263-269.

[6] C. Caldas, *et al.*, Detection of K-ras mutations in the stool of patients with pancreatic adenocarcinoma and pancreatic ductal hyperplasia. Cancer Res **54** (1994), 3568-3573.

[7] C. Caldas, *et al.*, Frequent somatic mutations and homozygous deletions of the p16 (MTS1) gene in pancreatic adenocarcinoma. Nature Genet **8** (1994), 27-32.

[8] S.A. Hahn, *et al.*, DPC4, a candidate tumor suppressor gene at human chromosome 18q21.1. Science **271** (1996), 350-353.

[9] S.A. Hahn, *et al.*, Allelotype of pancreatic adenocarcinoma using xenograft enrichment. Cancer Res **55** (1995), 4670-4675.

[10] A. Hoorens, *et al.*, Pancreatic acinar cell carcinoma. An analysis of cell lineage markers, p53 expression, and Ki-ras mutation. Am J Pathol **143** (1993), 685-698.

[11] R.H. Hruban, *et al.*, K-ras oncogene activation in adenocarcinoma of the human pancreas. A study of 82 carcinomas using a combination of mutant-enriched polymerase chain reaction analysis and allele-specific oligonucleotide hybridization. Am J Pathol **143** (1993), 545-554.

[12] H. Kalthoff, *et al.*, p53 and K-RAS alterations in pancreatic epithelial cell lesions. Oncogene **8** (1993), 289-298.
[13] P.G. Komarov, *et al.*, A chemical inhibitor of p53 that protects mice from the side effects of cancer therapy. Science **285** (1999), 1733-1737.
[14] H. Kondo, *et al.*, Detection of K-ras gene mutations at codon 12 in the pancreatic juice of patients with intraductal papillary mucinous tumors of the pancreas. Cancer **79** (1997), 900-905.
[15] K.Y. Lam and C.Y. Lo, Role of p53 tumor suppressor gene in pancreatic endocrine tumors of Chinese patients. Am J Gastroenterol **93** (1998), 1232-1235.
[16] W.Y. Lee, *et al.*, Papillary cystic tumors of the pancreas: assessment of malignant potential by analysis of progesterone receptor, flow cytometry, and ras oncogene mutation. Anticancer Res **17** (1997), 2587-2591.
[17] N.S. Pellegata, *et al.*, K-ras and p53 gene mutations in pancreatic cancer: ductal and nonductal tumors progress through different genetic lesions. Cancer Res **54** (1994), 1556-1560.
[18] M.S. Redston, *et al.*, p53 mutations in pancreatic carcinoma and evidence of common involvement of homocopolymer tracts in DNA microdeletions. Cancer Res **54** (1994), 3025-3033.
[19] E. Rozenblum, *et al.*, Tumor-suppressive pathways in pancreatic carcinoma. Cancer Res **57** (1997), 1731-1734.
[20] K. Satoh, *et al.*, K-ras mutation and p53 protein accumulation in intraductal mucin- hypersecreting neoplasms of the pancreas. Pancreas **12** (1996), 362-368.
[21] A. Scarpa, *et al.*, Pancreatic adenocarcinomas frequently show p53 gene mutations. Am J Pathol **142** (1993), 1534-1543.
[22] A. Scarpa, *et al.*, Pancreatic cancer in Europe: Ki-ras gene mutation pattern shows geographical differences. Int J Cancer **57** (1994), 167-171.
[23] M. Schutte, *et al.*, Abrogation of the Rb/p16 tumor-suppressive pathway in virtually all pancreatic carcinomas. Cancer Res **57** (1997), 3126-3130.
[24] M. Schutte, *et al.*, DPC4 gene in various tumor types. Cancer Res **56** (1996), 2527-2530.
[25] F. Sessa, *et al.*, Intraductal papillary-mucinous pancreatic tumors are phenotypically, genetically and behaviorally distinct growths. An analysis of tumor cell phenotype, K-ras and p53 gene mutations. Virchows Archiv **425** (1994), 357-367.
[26] V.T. Smit, *et al.*, KRAS codon 12 mutations occur very frequently in pancreatic adenocarcinomas. Nucleic Acids Res **16** (1988), 7773-7782.
[27] P.G. Terhune, *et al.*, Only wild-type c-Ki-ras codons 12, 13, and 61 in human pancreatic acinar cell carcinomas. Mol Carcinog **10** (1994), 110-114.
[28] A. Villanueva, *et al.*, Disruption of the antiproliferative TGF-beta signaling pathways in human pancreatic cancer cells. Oncogene **17** (1998), 1969-1978.
[29] K. Z'Graggen, *et al.*, Prevalence of activating K-ras mutations in the evolutionary stages of neoplasia in intraductal papillary mucinous tumors of the pancreas. Ann Surg **226** (1997), 491-498.

Part II: Expression studies in pancreatic cancer

Molecular Pathogenesis of Pancreatic Cancer
T.M. Gress (Ed.)
IOS Press, 2000

Application of suppression subtractive hybridisation for identification of genes regulated by the TF-FVIIa pathway in pancreatic cancer

T. Taniguchi and N. R. Lemoine
Imperial Cancer Research Fund Molecular Oncology Unit, Imperial College School of Medicine, Hammersmith Campus, DuCane Road, London W12 0NN, UK

The tissue factor (TF)/factor VIIa (FVIIa) complex initiates the coagulation cascade leading to thrombin generation and fibrin deposition. It has been also demonstrated that TF plays important roles in tumour invasion and metastasis. Previous work has shown an association between TF expression and histological grade of human cancers, including glioma [1], lung cancer [2], colorectal cancer [3], and pancreatic cancer [4]. We have utilised the suppression subtractive hybridisation technique in order to identify alterations in gene expression in human pancreatic cancer cell lines upon binding of FVIIa to TF. Sequence analysis revealed that nine out of 16 clones identified matched previous described genes in the Genbank/EMBL databases while the identities of the other seven are presently unknown. We have already confirmed that five genes were upregulated by the TF-FVIIa pathway by using northern blotting. This study provides new evidence that the TF-FVIIa pathway is implicated in upregulation of a number of important genes that can determine cell behaviour of cancer cells.

1. INTRODUCTION

TF is highly expressed in cancer cell lines which show enhanced metastatic potential and it is also involved in the regulation of tumour growth [5,6] Melanoma cells that highly express TF on their cell surface showed a higher frequency of lung metastasis than low TF-expressing cells in mice [5]. Functional inhibition of TF using an anti-TF antibody results in a significant reduction of the number of experimental pulmonary metastases in SCID mice [7]. The prometastatic function of TF was also shown on Chinese Hamster Ovary (CHO) cells transfected with TF [8]. In this experimental model, ligand binding of FVIIa to TF is required for metastasis, while binding of chemically inactivated FVIIa is antimetastatic. Thus, not only expression of TF on the cell surface but also binding of catalytically active FVIIa is necessary for tumour cell metastasis.

TF is also a member of the class II cytokine receptor superfamily, which includes the interferon (IFN) α/β and γ receptor, inducing an intracellular signal upon binding of its specific ligand FVII(a). Recently, it was reported that TF supports cell adhesion and migration through recruitment of actin-binding protein 280 (ABP-280, filamin 1) to TF-mediated adhesion sites [9]. Furthermore, replacement of TF's cytoplasmic Ser residues with Asp to mimic phosphorylation enhances interaction with ABP-280, whereas Ala mutations abolish coprecipitation of ABP-280 with the immobilised TF cytoplasmic domain, and severely reduce cell spreading. Our own data also suggest that signalling through the TF/FVIIa pathway is involved in specific upregulation of uPAR gene expression, resulting in enhanced invasive properties of cancer cells [10]. Inhibition of the TF/FVII(a) complex using genetic approaches to reduce TF expression or induce antagonist of FVII could be an attractive approaches to suppress the epithelial-stromal interactions which are critical to angiogenesis and tumour invasion. Therefore, TF initiates intracellular signalling that involves this or other factors that interact with the TF cytoplasmic domain.

2. RESULTS

We have utilised the suppression subtractive hybridisation technique in order to identify alterations in gene expression in human pancreatic cancer cell lines upon binding of FVIIa to TF.

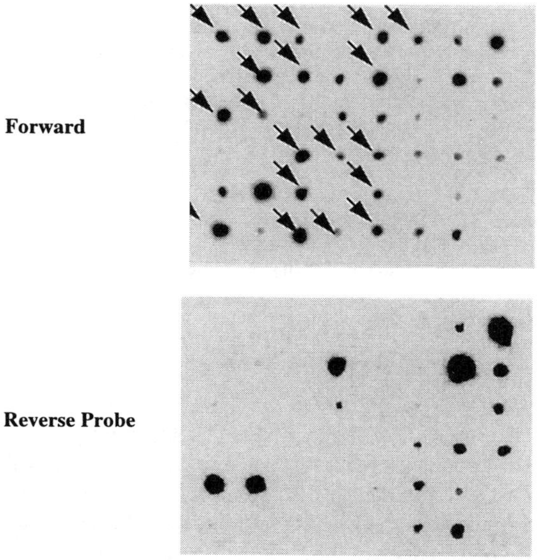

Figure 1 Differential screening of subtracted cDNAs using a cDNA array technique. The forward-subtracted experimental cDNA PCR product was subcloned into the pCR2.1-TOPO plasmid vector and transformed into TOP10 cells. PCR amplification showed that 46 out of 96 colonies contained cDNA inserts. The PCR products were spotted on two identical Hybond-N+ nylon membranes. Dot blots hybridised with cDNA probes made from forward-subtracted cDNA and reverse-subtracted cDNA. The arrows point to differentially expressed clones.

The forward-subtracted experimental cDNA PCR product was subcloned into the pCR2.1-TOPO plasmid vector and transformed into the TOP10 cells using the TOPO TA Cloning kit (Invitrogen). PCR revealed that 46 out of 96 colonies contained cDNA inserts ranging from approximately 150 bp to 1000 bp. Each PCR product was spotted on two identical Hybond-N+ nylon membranes and hybridised with radiolabelled forward- or reverse-subtracted cDNAs whose adaptor sequences were removed by restriction digestion. Nineteen clones showed positive after differential screening (Fig. 1). Sequence analysis revealed that nine out of these 16 clones matched previous described genes in the Genbank/EMBL databases while the identities of the other seven are presently unknown. We have already confirmed that five genes were upregulated by the TF-FVIIa pathway by using northern blotting.

3. DISCUSSION

This study provided new evidence that the TF-FVIIa pathway is implicated in upregulation of a number of important genes that can determine cell behaviour of cancer cells. However, further work is required to show how these series of genes upregulated through the TF-FVIIa pathway are orchestrated to influence cell fate and behaviour, such as cell proliferation or escape from apoptosis.

References

[1] K. Hamada *et al*, Expression of tissue factor correlates with grade of malignancy in human glioma, *Cancer* **77** (1996) 1877-83.

[2] M. Sawada *et al*, Expression of tissue factor in non-small-cell lung cancers and its relationship to metastasis, *British Journal of Cancer* **79** (1999) 472-7.

[3] H.Kataoka *et al*, Analysis of tissue factor and tissue factor pathway inhibitor expression in human colorectal carcinoma cell lines and metastatic sublines to the liver, *International Journal of Cancer* **72** (1997) 878-84.

[4] A.K. Kakkar *et al*, Tissue factor expression correlates with histological grade in human pancreatic cancer, *British Journal of Surgery* **82** (1995) 1101-4.

[5] B.M.Mueller *et al*, Expression of tissue factor by melanoma cells promotes efficient hematogenous metastasis, *Proceedings of National Academic Sciences USA* **89** (1992) 11832-6.

[6] M.E. Bromberg *et al*, Tissue factor promotes melanoma metastasis by a pathway independent of blood coagulation, *Proceedings National Academic Sciences USA* **92** (1995) 8205-9.

[7] E.G. Fischer *et al*, Tissue factor-initiated thrombin generation activates the signaling thrombin receptor on malignant melanoma cells, *Cancer Research* **55** (1995) 1629-32.

[8] B.M.Mueller *et al*, Requirement for binding of catalytically active factor VIIa in tissue factor-dependent experimental metastasis, *Journal of Clinical Investigation* **101** (1998) 1372-8.

[9] I Ott *et al*, A role for tissue factor in cell adhesion and migration mediated by interaction with actin-binding protein 280, *Journal of Cell Biology* **140** (1998) 1241-53.

[10] T. Taniguchi *et al*, Enhanced expression of urokinase receptor induced through the tissue factor-factor VIIa pathway in human pancreatic cancer, *Cancer Research* **58** (1998) 4461-7.

Molecular Pathogenesis of Pancreatic Cancer
T.M. Gress (Ed.)
IOS Press, 2000

The human homologue of the mouse *Rab20* gene is overexpressed in pancreatic carcinoma

J.M. Amillet[1], M. Muleris[1], F. Müller-Pillasch[2], T.M. Gress[2], G. Goubin[1]
1) UMR 147 CNRS, Institut Curie, 26 rue d'Ulm, 75248 Paris Cedex 05, France
2) Department of Internal Medizin I, Universitätsklinikum Ulm, 89081 Ulm, Germany

SUMMARY

A previous search for genes overexpressed in pancreatic cancer using gridded arrays of cDNA libraries and differential hybridization revealed about 400 cDNA clones. One of them is homologous to the mouse Rab20 cDNA. The Rab20 protein is a member of a large family of small GTPases which are specific regulators of vesicular transport. Northern blot analysis showed that RAB20 mRNA is restricted to certain tissues and overexpressed in more than 50% of the pancreatic cancer cell lines and 2 of 5 pancreatic carcinomas. By fluorescence *in situ* hybridization the human *RAB20* gene was assigned to the region qter of chromosome 13. High levels of expression of *RAB20* in pancreatic cancer cells suggest that a selective growth advantage may result from modifications of intracellular vesicular transport. However, the role of RAB20 in human tumor cells is unknown and remains to be elucidated.

INTRODUCTION

As part of a collaboration with the Department of Internal Medicine I of the University of Ulm we have undertaken the characterization of cDNA clones overexpressed in pancreatic cancer tissues. These clones were selected using gridded arrays of cDNA libraries and differential hybridization [1]. One of these clones, named xs17, is strongly homologous to the Rab20 cDNA of mouse. The Rab20 protein is a member of a large family of small GTPases which are specific and essential regulators of vesicular transport [2]. Rab proteins are localized on the cytoplasmic face of organelles and vesicles involved in the biosynthetic/secretory and endocytic pathways in eucaryotic cells [3, 4]. While Rab proteins have been identified in many eucaryotes, Rab20 has only been described in mouse [5]. In addition to be present in non-polarized cells Rab20 is mainly expressed in the apical domain of kidney tubule and intestine epithelial cells. Electron microscopic studies revealed that Rab20 is located in endocytic structures underlying the apical plasma membrane. This suggests that Rab20 is involved in apical endocytosis and membrane recycling in polarized cells.

RESULTS

Sequence of the human RAB20 protein

The complete sequence of the open reading frame was obtained by RACE-PCR. The deduced amino acid sequence displays 82% identity with the mouse protein without any gap in the alignment and with 13 conservative substitutions (Fig. 1). The N-terminal region is particularly well conserved between mouse and human. This supports the fact that we have isolated the human homologue of the mouse *Rab20* gene.

```
Human   1    MRKPDSKIVLLGDMNVGKTSLLQRYMERRFPDTVSTVGGAFYLKQWRSYNISIWDTAGRE
             MRKPD KIVLLGDMNVGKTSLLQRYMERRFPDTVSTVGGAFYLKQWRS+NISIWDTAGRE
Mouse   1    MRKPDGKIVLLGDMNVGKTSLLQRYMERRFPDTVSTVGGAFYLKQWRSFNISIWDTAGRE

Human   61   QFHGLGSMYCRGAAAIILTYDVNHRQSLVELEDRFLGLTDTASKDCLFAIVGNKVDLTEE
             QFHGLGS+YCRGAAAIILTYDVNH QSL ELEDRFLGLT+TA+ DCLFAIVGNKVDLT E
Mouse   61   QFHGLGSLYCRGAAAIILTYDVNHPQSLFELEDRFLGLTETANNDCLFAIVGNKVDLTSE

Human   121  GALAGQEKEECSPNMDAGDRVSPRAPKQVQLEDAVALYKKILKYKMLDEQDVPAAEQMCF
                 G EKE  +     G  VS + PKQVQ EDAVALYKKILKYKMLDE+++PAAEQMCF
Mouse   121  RDTEGGEKEGPASG-KVGSCVSTKVPKQVQPEDAVALYKKILKYKMLDEREMPAAEQMCF

Human   181  ETSAKTGYNVDLLFETLFDLVVPMILQQRAERPSHTVDISSHKPPKRTRSGCCA
             ETSAKTGYNVDLLFETLFDLVVPMI++QRAE    TVDI+S K PK+TRSGCCA
Mouse   180  ETSAKTGYNVDLLFETLFDLVVPMIMRQRAEESDQTVDIASCKTPKQTRSGCCA
```

Figure 1:
Amino acid sequences alignment of the human and mouse Rab20 proteins. The (+) indicates a conservative substitution.

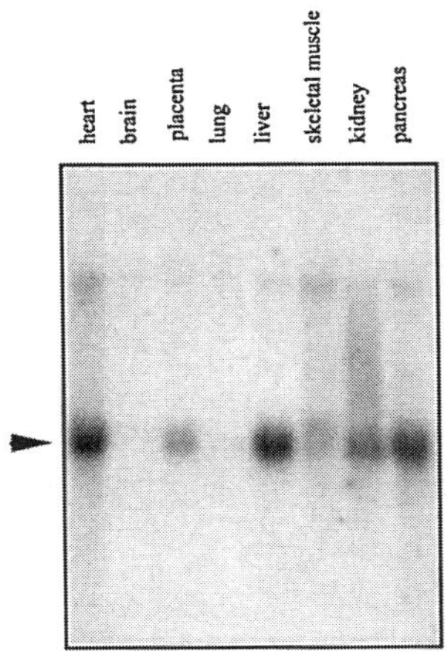

Figure 2:
RAB20 mRNA expression in human tissues. A commercially available northern blot (Clontech) containing 2 μg of polyA+ RNA from the indicated tissues was probed with the 1.2 kb insert of the xs17 plasmid.

RAB20 mRNA expression in human tissues

RAB20 mRNA expression was analysed in different human tissues by northern blot hybridization with polyA$^+$ RNA. As shown in Figure 2, the RAB20 transcript is mainly expressed in heart, liver and pancreas. Lower expression was observed in placenta, skeletal muscle and kidney whereas no signal was detected in brain and lung. Therefore the expression of RAB20 mRNA is restricted to certain tissues.

RAB20 mRNA expression in pancreatic cancer cell lines, pancreatic carcinoma, chronic pancreatitis and healthy pancreas

The expression of RAB20 mRNA was first analysed in pancreatic cancer cell lines. The RAB20 transcript was detected at moderate to high levels in 7 cell lines and was almost undetectable in 3 cell lines (Fig.3).
To determine whether RAB20 expression is altered in pancreatic tumors 5 samples of pancreatic carcinoma, chronic pancreatitis and healthy pancreas were analyzed by northern blot. The RAB20 transcript in healthy pancreas and chronic pancreatitis was not detected after 4-day exposure whereas in 2 of 5 pancreatic carcinomas a sharp signal was observed (data not shown). Therefore RAB20 is overexpressed in more than 50% of the pancreatic cancer cell lines and in 2 of 5 pancreatic carcinomas as compared to chronic pancreatitis and healthy pancreas.

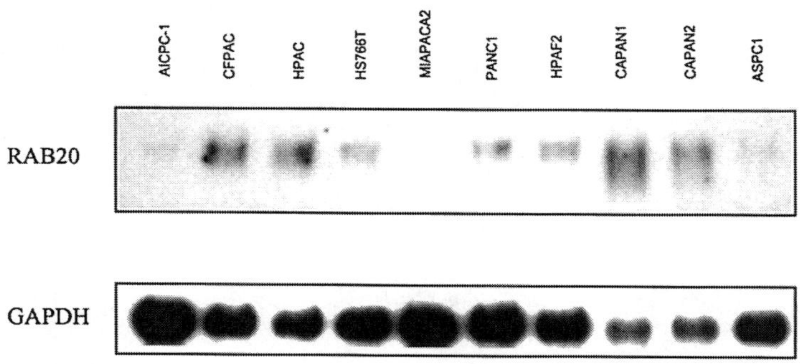

Figure 3:
RAB20 mRNA expression in pancreatic cancer cell lines. 10 µg of total RNA were probed with the 1.2 kb insert of the xs17 plasmid. The quantity and the amount of RNA loaded in each lane were controlled by hybridization with a GAPDH probe.

Chromosomal Localization

The chromosomal localization of the *RAB20* gene was determined by fluorescence *in situ* hybridization. The *RAB20* gene maps to the region qter of chromosome 13 (data not shown). No amplification of this region has been reported in pancreatic cancer.

DISCUSSION

The data presented in this report suggest that overexpression of the RAB20 protein is associated with initiation or progression of tumorigenesis in a subset of pancreatic carcinoma. However, additional samples should be analyzed to assess the precise frequency of overexpression and to search for an association with a particular subtype of carcinoma. Another gene implicated in the regulation of vesicular transport, *MSS4*, is also overexpressed in pancreatic cancer tissue [6]. This gene encodes a guanine-nucleotide-exchange factor for the RAB family [7]. Higher levels of expression of *RAB20* and *MSS4* in pancreatic cancer cells suggest that a selective growth advantage may result from modifications of intracellular vesicular transport. Several studies have shown that some RAB factors were implicated in the regulation of cell adhesion and migration. For instance, some RAB family members are involved in growth factors (HGF)-induced endocytosis and exocytosis of adhesion molecules such as integrin and cadherin [8]. Introduction of an activated Rab5 protein in fibroblasts also induced a reorganization of the actin cytoskeleton and cell migration [9]. In this context it will be of importance to analyse the effects of the overexpression of RAB20 on cell adhesion and migration.

REFERENCES

[1] Gress TM, Müller-Pillasch F, Geng M, Zimmerhackl F, Zehetner G, Friess H, Buchler M, Adler G, Lehrach H. A pancreatic cancer-specific expression profile. Oncogene (1996) **13**:1819-30.

[2] Zerial M, Stenmark H. Rab GTPases in vesicular transport. Curr Opin Cell Biol. (1993) **5**:613-20.

[3] Schimmoller F, Simon I, Pfeffer SR. Rab GTPases, directors of vesicle docking. J Biol Chem. (1998) **273**:22161-4.

[4] Gonzalez L Jr, Scheller RH. Regulation of membrane trafficking: structural insights from a Rab/effector complex. Cell (1999) **96**:755-8.

[5] Lutcke A, Parton RG, Murphy C, Olkkonen VM, Dupree P, Valencia A, Simons K, Zerial M. Cloning and subcellular localization of novel rab proteins reveals polarized and cell type-specific expression. J Cell Sci. (1994) **107**:3437-48.

[6] Müller-Pillasch F, Zimmerhackl F, Lacher U, Schultz N, Hameister H, Varga G, Friess H, Buchler M, Adler G, Gress TM. Cloning of novel transcripts of the human guanine-nucleotide-exchange factor Mss4: in situ chromosomal mapping and expression in pancreatic cancer. Genomics (1997) **46**:389-96.

[7] Yu H, Schreiber SL. Cloning, Zn2+ binding, and structural characterization of the guanine nucleotide exchange factor human Mss4. Biochemistry (1995) **34**:9103-10.

[8] Kamei T, Matozaki T, Takai Y. Mechanisms of cell adhesion and migration. Gan To Kagaku Ryoho (1999) **26**:1359-66.

[9] Spaargaren M, Bos JL. Rab5 induces Rac-independent lamellipodia formation and cell migration. Mol Biol Cell (1999) **10**:3239-50.

Molecular Pathogenesis of Pancreatic Cancer
T.M. Gress (Ed.)
IOS Press, 2000

Identification and characterisation of TGFβ1 target genes in the pancreatic cancer cell line PANC-1

V.Ellenrieder*, G. Sommer*, M.M.Geng, G.Adler, T.M. Gress
Department of Internal Medicine I, Universitätsklinikum Ulm, 89075 Ulm, Germany

The three mammalian TGFβ isoforms TGFβ1, TGFβ2 and TGFβ3 are homologous peptide growth regulatory factors, which act by binding to a single common receptor complex. TGFβ`s are implicated in multiple biological processes including embryogenesis, repair of soft and hard tissues, and regulation of hematopoiesis and of the immune response. Most importantly, the TGFβ`s are potent growth suppressors of many different normal cell types whereas, in contrast, many cancers are resistant to TGFβ. In sensitive cell types activities of TGFβ include induction of cell cycle arrest in late G1, induction of apoptosis, and induction of expression of cell adhesion molecules and components of the extracellular matrix, including fibronectin, laminin, collagen and integrins (for overviews see [1-3]). In the recent years TGFβ has been shown to be an important regulatory factor in rodent and human pancreas, in particular for the pathogenesis of inflammatory or malignant human pancreatic diseases. TGFβ is overexpressed in human chronic pancreatitis, and suggested to be involved in the pathogenesis of this chronic inflammtory disease of the pancreas [4]. In a number of animal models we and others could show that TGFβ is of paramount importance for the development of pancreatic fibrosis (see [5] for a review). TGFβ and TGFβRII [6, 7] have been described to be overexpressed in pancreatic cancer, but the functional significance of this overexpression is still mostly a matter of speculation.

Though the central role of TGFβ in pancreatic fibrosis and pancreatic cancer is well acknowledged, very little is known about TGFβ regulated target genes responsible for the morphological/phenotypic alterations induced by this growth factor in pancreatic cancer cells. In the present study we used the pancreatic cancer cell line PANC-1 to identify TGFβ target genes. For this purpose, we used arrays of cDNA clones previously isolated as differentially expressed in pancreatic cancer [8-10]. These cDNA clone arrays were hybridised with cDNA probes from PANC-1 cells enriched for TGFβ-regulated genes. For this purpose the cDNA-RDA method (representational difference analysis) [9-12] was modified to allow the generation of subtracted probes enriched for TGFβ target genes. The protocol was optimized to achieve a high specificity and to allow an easy interpretation of hybridisation results without the necessity to use expensive image analysis systems. Using this modified protocol we could describe for the first time the effect of TGFβ treatment on the "transcriptional phenotype" of pancreatic cancer cells with a functional TGFβ pathway.

---

* G.S. and V.E. contributed equally to this manuscript an should both be considered first authors.

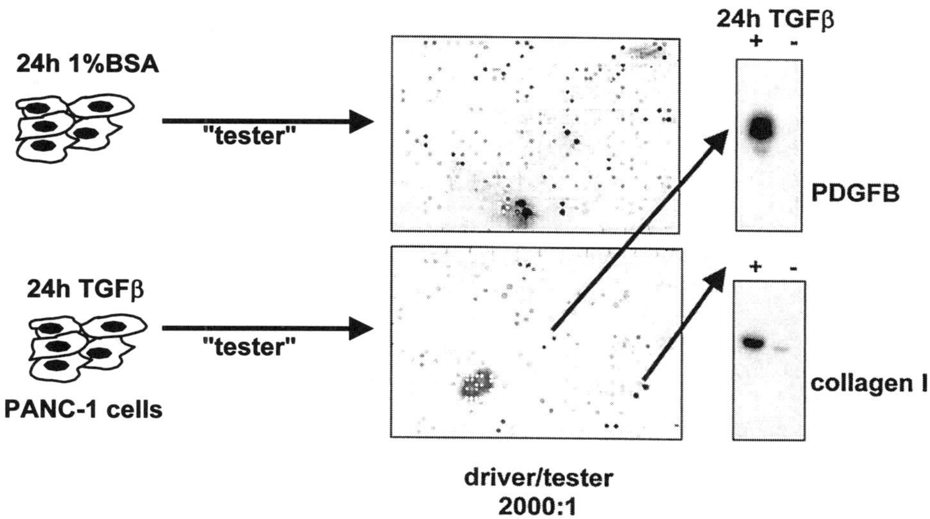

Figure 1

This figure summarizes the experimental approach used to identify TGFβ target genes in the pancreatic cancer cell line PANC-1. PANC-1 cells were treated with TGFβ (10ng/ml) for 24h, PANC-1 cells incubated for 24h in 1%BSA were used as control. In the RDA experiment mRNA from TGFβ-treated PANC-1 cells was used either as tester (to isolate upregulated genes) or driver (to isolate downregulated genes). The DP2-product obtained at a driver/tester ratio of 2000:1 was used for hybridisations with in-situ clone arrays containing around 500 genes isolated in previous approaches as differentially expressed in pancreatic cancer [8-10]. Northern blots containing 15 μg of total RNA from TGFβ-treated and untreated PANC-1 cells confirming the RDA-results are shown for a selection of genes [12].

TGFβ treatment led to an upregulation of genes involved in extracellular matrix composition and remodelling, including components of the extracellular matrix, such as collagen type I, the small proteoglycan biglycan [13] and the TGFβ-induced gene H3 (BGH3). BGH3 was cloned as TGFβ1-inducible gene from a human lung adenocarcinoma cell line [14]. It codes for a secreted protein with an RGD-binding site at its carboxyterminal end which appears to play a role in cell adhesion [15]. In addition, TGFβ may influence extracellular matrix formation by stimulating the growth of stromal fibroblasts. The growth stimulatory effect of TGFβ on fibroblasts has been attributed to the induction of PDGF, which has been shown by us in the present study and by other groups [16]. The TGFβ-treatment also induced transcripts for *MMP2*, a gelatinase showing a strong association with the metastatic potential of tumor cells [17]. In addition it induced transcripts for the plasminogen activator inhibitor [18] and reduced the transcript levels for bikunin/KOP (kunitz type plasmin inhibitor overexpressed in pancreatic cancer) [19]. Both proteins are important for inhibiting plasmin or plasminogen activation, and may thus participate in extracellular matrix turnover or in modulating the metastatic and invasive potential of tumor cells. Genes showing reduced transcript levels after a 24h treatment with TGFβ could be classified into two major groups. These included genes involved in transcriptional or translational regulation, as e.g,. *hnRNPc* [20], high mobility group protein *HMGI* (isoform Y, [21]), nuclear factor *NF45* [22] and the protein synthesis initiation factor EIF4 A-II [23]. Without going into the details of each individual gene we would interpret these alterations as markers of the inhibition of proliferation by TGFβ. Indeed we could show that a 24h treatment with TGFβ induces approximately 20% inhibition of proliferation of PANC-1 cells. The second major group included cytokeratins 7, 8, and 19, which are known markers of epithelial differentiation in the pancreas [24].

One of the most interesting TGFβ-target genes isolated in this approach, was biglycan. Biglycan (PG-I) belongs to the family of small leucine rich proteoglycans (SLRPs). This family comprises at least nine members, grouped together on the basis of their presence in the extracellular matrix and their leucine rich repeat domain that characterizes the structure of the protein core. The sequence of the core protein has been found in a variety of proteins throughout evolution and appears to be used for protein-protein, protein-cell or cell-cell interaction [25]. SLRPs are prominent constituents of the extracellular matrix (ECM). Biglycan was found cell surface associated in a variety of cell types, including epidermal cells, kidney collecting tube epithelial cells, blood vessel endothelial cells, myofibroblasts of the testis, chondrocytes and others. The ECM plays an integral role in development, tissue repair and metastasis. The SLRPs including biglycan appear to modulate these processes by regulation of matrix assembly, adhesion, migration and cellular growth. The pericellular localisation of biglycan as well as its ability to bind fibronectin suggest, that biglycan interferes with cell adhesion [26, 27]. Furthermore it may be associated with cell migration by influencing interactions of cell surface receptors with their matrix ligands [28, 29]. Interestingly SLRPs appear to participate in regulating the availability and function of growth factors such as TGFβ. TGFβ led to a strong induction of biglycan transcripts starting 8h and reaching maximal values 24h after treatment of PANC-1 cells. This effect was restricted to the cell line PANC-1 known to be responsive to TGFβ, whereas it could not be demonstrated in pancreatic cancer cell lines with a defective TGFβ pathway.

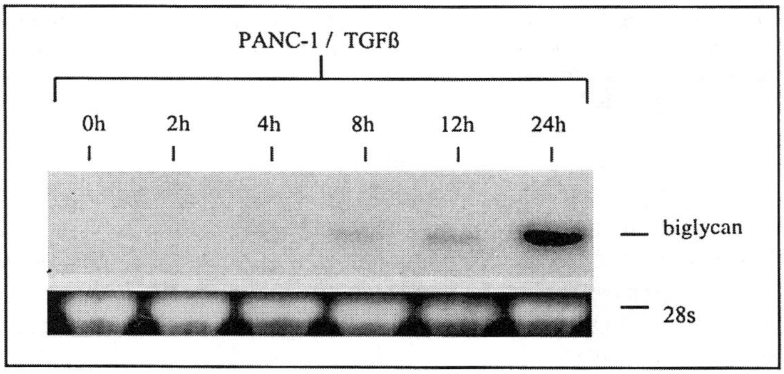

Figure 2

Time course of biglycan expression in PANC-1 cells after treatment with 10 ng/ml TGFβ. Northern blot analysis (20 μg total RNA per lane) revealed that upregulation of biglycan expression started after 8h and reached maximal values after 24 h.

This intriguing result led us to study the expression of biglycan in-vivo in human pancreatic tissues. Biglycan was strongly overexpressed in the majority of pancreatic cancer tissue samples as compared to normal pancreas. Elevated transcript levels were as well found in chronic pancreatitis tissue samples, though at much lower level as in pancreatic cancer tissues. There was no constitutive biglycan expression in all studied pancreatic cancer cell lines, whereas nude mouse xenografts of the same cell lines showed a strong biglycan expression localised to the stroma. Thus, in pancreatic cancer tissues the SLRP biglycan is strongly overexpressed and stromal cells appear to be its major source. Only pancreatic cancer cells with a functional TGFβ pathway appear to contribute to biglycan production in the presence of TGFβ. The known functions of biglycan as modulator of the ECM and the present data suggest, that biglycan may play a role in the development of the desmoplastic reaction in pancreatic cancer.

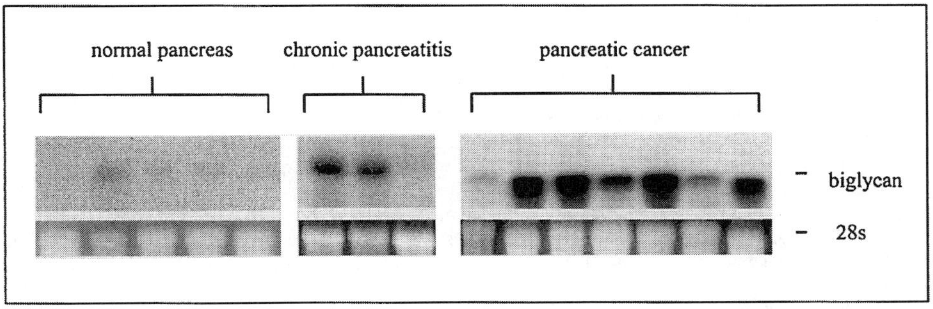

Figure 3
Biglycan mRNA expression in different pancreatic tissues was studied by Northern blot analysis (20 μg/ml total RNA per lane). Only a weak expression could be detected in normal pancreas tissue samples. Biglycan transcript levels were moderately eleveated in some chronic pancreatitis tissues samples, whereas and a strong overexpression was observed in the majority of the pancreatic cancer tissue samples.

To summarize, although our results certainly do not include all changes of gene expression occurring in pancreatic cancer cells upon treatment with TGFβ, they provide a good impression on the phenotypic plasticity induced by TGFβ in pancreatic cancer cells. Upon 24h of treatment with TGFβ PANC-1 cells gain characteristics usually attributed to fibroblasts as for example the synthesis of extracellular matrix components, *CTGF* or *MMP2*. In contrast, besides showing alterations indicative of the inhibition of proliferation, PANC-1 cells lose markers of epithelial differentiation. Thus, prolonged treatment with TGFβ appears to induce an epithelial-mesenchymal transdifferentiation of responsive pancreatic cancer cells. This is confirmed by the spindle-shaped morphology observed for PANC-1 cells after TGFβ treatment. Among others, this study has identified the small proteoglycan biglycan as a possible mediator of TGFβ actions on the ECM in pancreatic cancer. Biglycan may thus be involved in the development of the strong desmoplastic reaction usually observed in pancreatic tumours.

Acknowledgements

This work was supported in part by grants from the European Union (BMH4-CT98-3085) and the Deutsche Forschungsgemeinschaft (SFB518, Projects B1 and C1) to TMG.

References

[1] J. Massague, TGF-beta signal transduction. Annu Rev Biochem.**67**(1998) 753-91.

[2] M. Kretzschmar amd J. Massague, SMADs: mediators and regulators of TGF-beta signaling. Curr Opin Genet Dev. **8** (1998) 103-11.

[3] S.D. Markowitz and A.B.Roberts, 1996. Tumour suppressor activity of the TGF-beta pathway in human cancers. Cytokine Growth Factor Rev. **7** (1996) 93-102.

[4] J.L.Van Laethem *et al*, Localization of transforming growth factor beta 1 and its latent binding protein in human chronic pancreatitis. Gastroenterology **108** (1995)1873-1881.

[5] T.M.Gress *et al*, Role of extracellular matrix in pancreatic diseases. Digestion **59** (1998) 625-637.

[6] H. Friess *et al*, Enhanced expression of the type II transforming growth factor beta receptor in human pancreatic cancer cells without alteration of type III receptor expression. Cancer Res **53** (1993) 2704-2707.

[7] H.Friess *et al*, Enhanced expression of transforming growth factor beta isoforms in pancreatic cancer correlates with decreased survival. Gastroenterology **105** (1993)1846-1856.
[8] T.M. Gress *et al*, A pancreatic cancer-specific expression profile. Oncogene **13** (1996) 1819-1830.
[9] T.M.Gress et al, Identification of genes with specific expression in pancreatic cancer by cDNA representational difference analysis. Genes Chromosomes Cancer **19** (1997) 97-103
[10] M.M. Geng *et a*l, Isolation of differentially expressed genes by combining representational difference analysis (RDA) and cDNA library arrays. BioTechniques **25/3** (1998) 434-438.
[11] M. Hubank and D.G. Schatz, Identifying differences in mRNA expression by representational difference analysis of cDNA. Nucleic Acids Res **22** (1994) 5640-5648.
[12] M.M.Geng *et al*, Use of representational difference analysis to study the effect of TGFβ on the expression profile of a pancreatic cancer cell line. Genes Chromosom. Cancer **26** (1999) 70-79.
[13] M.A. Haralson and JR Hassel, The extracellular matrix- an overview. In Haralson MA, Hassel JR, editors. Extracellular matrix. Oxford: Oxford University press, 1-30, 1995.
[14] J.Skonier *et al*, cDNA cloning and sequence analysis of beta ig-h3, a novel gene induced in a human adenocarcinoma cell line after treatment with transforming growth factor-beta. DNA Cell Biol **11** (1992) 511-522.
[15] J.Skonier *et al*, beta ig-h3: a transforming growth factor-beta-responsive gene encoding a secreted protein that inhibits cell attachment in vitro and suppresses the growth of CHO cells in nude mice. DNA Cell Biol **13** (1994) 571-584.
[16] M. Ebert *et al*, Induction of platelet-derived growth factor A and B chains and over-expression of their receptors in human pancreatic cancer. Int J Cancer 62 (1995) 529-535.
[17] S.M.Krane, Clinical importance of metalloproteinases and their inhibitors. Ann N Y Acad Sci **732** (1994) 1-10.
[18] C.W.Crowley *et al*, 1993. Prevention of metastasis by inhibition of the urokinase receptor. Proc Natl Acad Sci U S A **90** (1993) 5021-5025.
[19] F.Müller Pillasch *et al*, Cloning of a new Kunitz-type protease inhibitor with a putative transmembrane domain overexpressed in pancreatic cancer. Biochim Biophys Acta **1395** (1998) 88-95.
[20] C.G.Burd *et al*,. Primary structures of the heterogeneous nuclear ribonucleoprotein A2, B1, and C2 proteins: a diversity of RNA binding proteins is generated by small peptide inserts. Proc Natl Acad Sci USA **86** (1989) 9788-9792.
[21] R.Reeves and M.S. Nissen, Cell cycle regulation and functions of HMG-I(Y). Prog Cell Cycle Res **1** (1995) 339-349.
[22] P.N. Kao *et al*, Cloning and expression of cyclosporin A- and FK506-sensitive nuclear factor of activated T-cells: NF45 and NF90. J Biol Chem **269** (1994) 20691-20699.
[23] K. Sudo *et al*, Isolation and mapping of the human EIF4A2 gene homologous to the murine protein synthesis initiation factor 4A-II gene Eif4a2. Cytogenet Cell Genet **71** (1995) 385-388.
[24] M.R. Vila *et al*, Cytokeratins and mucins as molecular markers of cell differentiation and neoplastic transformation in the exocrine pancreas. Zentralbl Pathol **140** (1994) 225-235.
[25] S. Henikoff *et al*, Gene families: the taxonomy of protein paralogs and chimeras. Science **278** (1997) 609-614.
[26] R. Fleischmajer *et al*, Decorin interacts with fibrillar collagen of embryonic and adult human skin. J.Struct.Biol. **106** (1991) 82-90;
[27] D. Bidanset *et al*, Regulation of cell substrate adhesion: effects of small galactosaminoglycan-containing proteoglycans J.Cell Biol **118** (1992) 1523-1531
[28] M. Kinsella , Selective expression and processing of biglycan during migration of bovine aortic endothelial cells. Thhe role of endogeneous fibroblast growth factor J.Biol.Chem. **272** (1997) 318-325.
[29] J.Couchman, Distribution of two basement membrane proteoglycans through hair follicle development and the hair growth cycle in the rat. J.Invest.Dermatol. **94** (1990) 7s-14s.

Expression of regulatory peptide receptors in pancreatic cancer cell lines

B. Burghardt[1], G. Rácz[1], L. Flautner[2], T.M. Gress[3], G. Varga[1]
[1]*Institute of Experimental Medicine, Hungarian Academy of Sciences, 1083 Budapest, Hungary* [2]*1st Department of Surgery, Semmelweis University, 1083 Budapest, Hungary*
[3]*Department of Internal Medizin I, University of Ulm, 89081 Ulm, Germany*

An important role for regulatory peptides, such as the members of the CCK peptide family and somatostatin, in tumors of the pancreas is supported by a number of recent observations. These peptides have been shown to either stimulate or inhibit mitogenesis by receptor-mediated mechanisms [1]. Furthermore, the receptors for these peptides belong to the family of G-protein-coupled receptors. There is evidence that alterations in G-protein-coupled signal-transduction pathways are involved in modulating protooncogene and tumor suppressor gene expression [1]. In several cell lines, cholecystokinin/gastrin-like peptides have been shown to be autocrine regulators of cell proliferation [2, 3]. Somatostatin, however, inhibits cell proliferation not only in pancreatic cell lines but also in certain cases of human pancreatic cancer [1, 3].

In the present work we sought for the presence of CCK-A and CCK-B, as well as somatostatin-2 (SSTR2) receptors on several well-characterized cell lines originating from pancreatic adenocarcinoma. We also studied the effects of CCK and the somatostatin analogue octreotide on DNA synthesis in these cells. Capan-1, Capan-2, Panc-1, MiaPaca-2, HPAF human pancreatic adenocarcinoma cell lines, as well as CCK-A receptor- and CCK-B receptor-transfected Panc-1 cells were used. Transfected Panc-1 cells were kindly provided by Dr. Craig Logsdon (Univ. Michigan, Ann Arbor, MI). The expression of SSTR2, CCK-A and CCK-B receptor mRNA in these cell lines was shown by reverse transcriptase-polymerase chain reaction (RT-PCR). Cultured cells were grown in 75 cm^2 flasks and directly lysed in RNA-Clean solution (AGS GmbH, Heidelberg, Germany). Total RNA was extracted according to the manufacturer's instructions. To remove DNA contamination, 10 μg total RNA was treated with 10 U Rnase-free Dnase-I (Boehringer Mannheim) in a PE buffer containing 78 U RNasin (Promega, Germany) at room temperature for 30 min in a final volume of 50 μl. After phenol, phenol/$CHCl_3$/IAA and $CHCl_3$/IAA extraction the RNA was precipitated, centrifuged and dried. Reverse transcription was then carried out in 50 mM Tris-HCl buffer (pH 8.3) containing 75 mM KCl, 3mM $MgCl_2$, 10mM DTT, 0.5 mM of each dNTP, 0.5 μg oligo d(T) and the RNA pellet in a final volume of 20 μl. After a 2-min incubation at 42°C, 200 U reverse transcriptase (SuperScript II, Gibco Laboratories) was added to the reverse transcription mixture which was then incubated for 50 min at 42°C, followed by 15 min at 70°C. 1μl cDNA was used for amplification. PCR reaction was performed in a final volume of 50 μl containing 1 μl cDNA, 5 or 2.5 U of Taq polymerase (Sigma, St. Louis, MO), using specific sense and antisense primers (100 mM of SSTR2, CCK-AR, CCK-BR and 250 mM of human acidic ribosomal phosphoprotein), and 200 μM deoxynucleotide triphosphate in 10 mM Tris-HCl buffer (pH=9) containing 1.5 mM $MgCl_2$, 50 mM KCl, and 0.01 % Triton X-100.

Following denaturation of the samples at 94°C for 3 min, the PCR reactions were carried out on a DNA Thermal Cycler (Hybaid). To identify SSTR2 35 cycle reaction was performed for 30 sec at 94°C (denaturation), for 1 min at 58°C (annealing), for 2 min at 72°C (extension) using primers 5'-ATGGACATGGCGGATGAGCCACT-3', and 5'-TACTGGTTTGGAGGTCTCCATTGA-3'). To amplify CCK-A receptor mRNA 30 cycle reaction was performed for 30 sec at 94°C, for 30 sec at 55°C, for 1 min at 72°C using primers 5'-ATGATGGTGGCATATGGATTAATCTCTTTGG-3', 5'-TGTAGGACAGGAGG-AGGATGAAGGAAAT-3'). To investigate the presence of CCK-B receptors 35 cycle reaction was performed for 45 sec at 94°C, for 30 sec at 55°C, for 1 min at 72°C using primers 5'-GTGGCCTACGGG-CTTATCTCTCGCGAGCTCTACTTA-3' and 5'-ACGTGTTGGCACTATAAA-CTGGCAACCAACACAG-3'). Human acidic ribosomal phosphoprotein was used as an internal control since it was previously shown to be expressed at the same level in both normal, inflamed, and malignant pancreatic tissues [4]. Primers of human acidic ribosomal protein were 5'-CTGGCTAAGTTGGTTGCTTT-3' and 5'-GCAGCTGATCAAGACTGGA-3'; 19 cycles, denaturating at 94°C for 30 sec, annealing at 58°C for 1 min, extension at 72°C for 2 min. The amplification was terminated by a final extension step at 72°C for 10 min in all cases. RT-PCR products were analyzed by electrophoresis on a 1.5 % agarose gel, stained with ethidium bromide and exposed to UV light.

Cells were maintained at 37°C in a humidified atmosphere of 5% CO_2 and 95% air in DMEM medium supplemented with 10 percent fetal calf serum (FCS). In each experiment, the cells were first incubated in serum-free DMEM containing 0.2% bovine serum albumin (BSA) for 24 h. The cells were then treated with 10 percent FCS, octreotide, CCK or the combination of one of the peptides with FCS. [^{3}H]thymidine incorporation into DNA was measured after either 24 h or 48 h incubation. Data are given as percent of [^{3}H]thymidine incorporation into untreated control cells from the same cell line.

RNA was extracted from human pancreatic adenocarcinoma cell lines and subjected to RT followed by PCR amplification. Human acidic ribosomal phosphoprotein was found to be expressed in both cell lines at similar levels (data not shown). Results of the PCR reaction revealed the presence of SSTR2 (1105 bp) PCR product in Capan-1, Capan-2, Miapaca-2 and HPAF cell lines (**Figure 1A**) but not in Panc-1 cells.

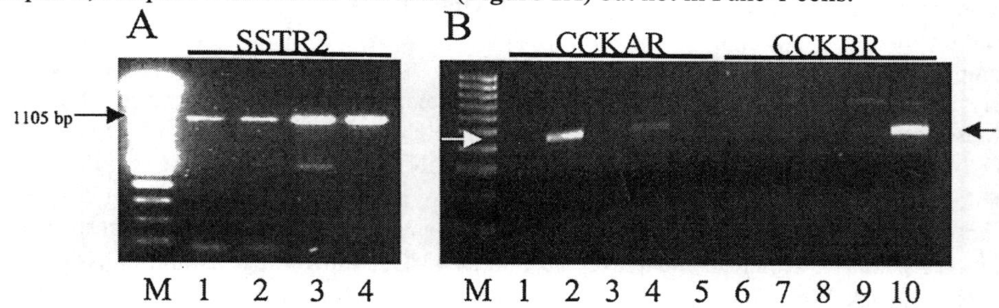

Figure 1. Detection of the presence of somatostatin-2 (SSTR2), CCK-A and CCK-B receptors in pancreatic cancer cell lines by RT-PCR. **Part A** shows RT-PCR for SSTR2 receptors. M: 100 bp ladder; cell lines: 1 MiaPaca, 2 Capan-1, 3 Capan-2, 4 HPAF cells. **Part B** shows RT-PCR for CCK-A and -B receptors. M: marker; cell lines: 1 Panc-1, 2 CCKAR-transfected Panc-1, 3 MiaPaCa, 4 CCKAR-transfected MiaPaCa, 5 CCKBR-transfected MiaPaCa, 6 Panc-1, 7 CCKAR-transfected Panc-1, 8 MiaPaCa, 9 CCKAR-transfected MiaPaCa, 10 CCKBR-transfected MiaPaCa cells.

No PCR products were obtained when CCK-A receptor and CCK-B receptor primers were used to amplify these receptors (data not shown) in any of the wild-type Capan-1, Capan-2, Panc-1, HPAF, Miapaca-2, and Panc-1 cells. On the contrary in CCK-A receptor transfected Panc-1 and Miapaca-2 cells PCR reaction yielded a 455 bp product corresponding to the expected size (**Figure 1B**). Similarly, following stable transfection, the PCR product corresponding to the CCK-B receptor mRNA was also detected (**Figure 1B**).

The growth-modulating effects of FCS and octreotide were investigated in Capan-2 and MiaPaca-2 cells. DNA synthesis in these cells, evaluated by [^{3}H]thymidine incorporation, was found to be stimulated by 10 percent FCS (**Table 1**). Octreotide significantly inhibited DNA synthesis. (**Table 1**). Compared to FCS treatment alone, the increase in [^{3}H]thymidine incorporation was significantly lower when FCS treatment was combined with octreotide in both cell lines (**Table 1**). CCK did not significantly modify the DNA synthesis in Capan-2, Miapaca and wild-type Panc-1 cells. In stably-transfected Panc-1 cells, however, the peptide induced a substantial, significant decrease in otherwise untreated and in FCS treated cells (**Table 2**).

Table 1
Rate of DNA synthesis in response to somatostatin analogue octreotide in Capan-2 and MiaPaca-2 cells. Values are given as ^{3}H-thymidine incorporation into DNA as a percent of control (48h exposure)

Cell line	Treatment	%	SEM	Difference
Capan-2	Oct	83.3	4.2	p<0.05 vs control
	FCS	130.4	5.4	p<0.05 vs control
	FCS+Oct	112.5	6.3	p<0.05 vs FCS alone
Miapaca2	Oct	81.4	3.5	p<0.05 vs control
	FCS	150.0	5.0	p<0.05 vs control
	FCS+Oct	117.5	3.3	p<0.05 vs FCS alone

FCS = 10 % fetal calf serum
oct = octreotide

Table 2
Rate of DNA synthesis in response to CCK in pancreatic adenocarcinoma cell lines. Values are given as ^{3}H-thymidine incorporation into DNA as a percent of control (24h exposure)

Cell line	Treatment	%	SEM	Difference
Capan-2	CCK	103.7	3.9	NS
Miapaca2	CCK	103.9	10.7	NS
Panc1	CCK	97.7	2.1	NS
Panc-1-tr*	CCK	25.6	2.0	p<0.05 vs control
	FCS	209.4	12.6	p<0.05 vs control
	FCS+CCK	55.0	8.9	p<0.05 vs FCS alone

*Panc-1-tr = CCK-A receptor-transfected Panc-1 cells
FCS = 10 % fetal calf serum

Recent studies suggest that several receptor types of somatostatin are present in normal human pancreas [5]. Among these receptors SSTR2 is thought to be responsible for mediating the antiproliferative effects [6]. Evidence was provided that one of the important signal-transduction pathways that is related to its suppressing effect on cell division is the stimulatory effect of somatostatin on intracellular phosphotyrosine phosphatase activity during activation of SSTR2 receptors [7]. Although type-2 somatostatin receptors are present in normal human tissues, as in the pancreas, colon and prostate, their expression is decreased or eliminated in advanced pancreatic and colorectal carcinomas as well as in prostate cancer [8, 9, 10, 11]. The loss of SSTR2 expression in tissues could represent a growth advantage for tumor cells and may explain the lack of antiproliferative effect of somatostatin analogue therapy on advanced carcinomas [10, 11]. Indeed, in human pancreatic carcinoma cell lines the restoration of SSTR2 receptor by stable transfection led to a significant reduction in cell growth and tumorigenicity [12]. All these findings suggest a central role of SSTR2 mediated processes in controlling cell proliferation not only in normal human pancreas but also in pancreatic adenocarcinoma. Therefore, it seems to be very important to characterize the proliferative effects and also the signal-transduction pathways coupled to these receptors. Previous studies variably reported the presence or absence of somatostatin receptors in pancreatic adenocarcinoma cell lines, depending on the cell line, and on the experimental conditions [8, 12]. In the present study we found that Capan-1, Capan-2 and Miapaca-2 cells express SSTR2 receptors. Our data therefore suggest that these cell lines are useful tools to study SSTR2-mediated processes. In accordance with the presence of SSTR2, octreotide, a somatostatin agonist that preferentially binds to type 2 somatostatin receptors [13], inhibited the proliferation of Capan-2 cells. Octreotide was able to inhibit the stimulatory action of serum addition into the medium. Previous work also showed that somatostatin and its analogues were able to inhibit cell proliferation in MiaPaca-2 cells [14], another cell line that express SSTR2 receptors detected both in the present and previous [12, 7] studies.

The available data about the presence of CCK receptors in human pancreas and pancreatic cancer cell lines are rather controversial. The expression of CCK-B receptors was detected in both normal and transformed pancreatic tissues [15, 16]. One study suggested that CCK-A receptors were also located in this organ [15]. Another one showed, however, that these receptors were expressed selectively in pancreatic adenocarcinomas but not in any normal specimens of this organ [16]. In fact the authors of the latter paper suggested that CCK-A receptor might serve as a selective biomarker of pancreatic adenocarcinoma because of its selective expression [16]. A series of studies from one laboratory reported that CCK stimulates the growth of several pancreatic adenocarcinoma cell lines, including MiaPaca-2, Panc-1 and Capan-2 [17, 18, 19]. These studies indicated that the stimulatory effect of CCK on Panc-1 cell line was mediated by CCK-B receptors [19]. Other investigators, however, could not confirm these findings. Native MiaPaca-2 and Panc-1 cells were reported not to possess CCK-A or CCK-B receptors by several investigations [20, 21, 22]. In the present study we found that neither CCK-A nor CCK-B receptors were expressed in native Capan-2, MiaPaca-2 and Panc-1 cells. In a similar manner, we found that these cells did not exhibit a proliferative response to CCK stimulation under our experimental conditions. Therefore, our observation is in line with those who could not find either CCK-A or CCK-B receptors, and did not observe CCK-mediated proliferative activities in human pancreatic carcinoma cell lines. We could confirm, however, the observation of Logsdon and coworkers [22] who found a very strong inhibitory effect of CCK in Panc-1 cells transfected with CCK-A receptors.

In conclusion, we found pancreatic adenocarcinoma cell lines that express functional SSTR2 receptors. However, among the cell lines investigated, no native cell lines expressed CCK-A and CCK-B receptors, and only CCK-A receptor-transfected cells responded to CCK with a modified proliferative response. The cell lines expressing peptide receptors and affecting DNA synthesis will serve as useful tools in further studies on gene expressional changes underlying G-protein activation induced inhibition of cell growth.

References

[1] N. Vaysse *et al*, Gastrointestinal peptides and receptors in pancreatic cancer In: Pancreatic cancer, molecular and clinical advances. (Neoptolemos JP, Lemoine NR eds) (1996) Blackwell, Oxford, 61-7

[2] G.S. Baldwin *et al*, The role of gastrin and cholecystokinin in normal and neoplastic gastrointestinal growth. J Gastroenterol Hepatol **10** (1995) 215-32

[3] M.L. Frazier *et al*, In: The pancreas: biology, pathobiology and disease. 2nd ed.(Go VLW *et al.*, eds.) (1993) Raven, New York, 565-73

[4] C. Wallrapp *et al*, Characterization of a high copy number amplification at 6q24 in pancreatic cancer indentities c-myb as a candidate oncogene. Cancer Research **57** (1997) 3135-3139

[5] Y.C. Patel *et al*, Subtype selectivity of peptide analogs for all five cloned human somatostatin receptors (hsstr 1-5). Endocrinology **135** (1994) 2814-2817

[6] L. Buscail *et al*, Inhibition of cell proliferation by the sometostatin analogue RC-160 is mediated by somatostatin receptor subtypes SSTR2 and SSTR5 through different mechanisms. Proc Natl Acad Sci USA **92** (1995) 1580-1584

[7] L. Buscail *et al*, Stimulation of tyrosine phosphatase and inhibition of cell proliferation by somatostatin analogues: Mediation by human somatostatin receptor subtypes SSTR1 and SSTR2. Proc Nat Acad Sci USA **91** (1994) 2315-2319

[8] L. Buscail *et al*, Loss of sst2 somatostatin receptor gene in human pancreatic and colorectal cancer. Cancer Res **56** (1996) 1823-1827

[9] J.C. Reubi *et al*, Somatostatin receptors in human prostate cancer. J Clin Endocrinol Metab **80** (1995) 2806-2814

[10] W.E. Fisher *et al*, Expression of the somatostatin receptor subtype-2 gene predicts response of human pancreatic cancer to octreotide. Surgery 120 (1996) 234-240

[11] C. Tang *et al*, Expression of somatostatin receptors in human pancreatic tumor. Pancreas **17** (1998) 80-84

[12] N. Delesque *et al*, Sst2 somatostatin receptor expression reverses tumorigenicity of human pancreatic cancer cells. Cancer Res **57** (1997) 956-962

[13] C. Bruns *et al*, Molecular pharmacology of somatostatin receptor subtypes. Ann NY Acad Sci **733** (1994) 138-146

[14] C. Liebow *et al*, Somatostatin analogues that inhibit growth of pancreatic cancer by stimulating tyrosin phosphatase. Proc Natl Acad Sci USA **86** (1989) 2003-2007

[15] H.J. Monstein *et al*, Cholecystokinin-A and Cholecystokinin-B/gastrin receptor mRNA expression in the gastrointestinal tract and pancreas of the rat and man. Scand J Gastroenterol **31** (1996) 383-390

[16] D.S. Weinberg *et al*, Cholecystokinin A and B receptors are differentially expressed in normal pancreas and pancreatic adenocarcinoma. J Clin Invest **100** (1997) 597-603

[17] J.P. Smith *et al*, Cholecystokinin stimulates growth of human pancreatic adenocarcinoma SW-1990. Dig Dis Sci **35** (1990) 1377-1384

[18] J.P. Smith *et al*, CCK stimulates growth of six human pancreatic cell lines in serum-free medium. Reg Peptides **32** (1991) 341-349

[19] J.P. Smith *et al*, Cholecystokinin receptors and PANC-1 human pancreatic cancer cells. Am J Physiol **265** (1993) G149-G155

[20] R.M. Liehr *et al*, Growth effects of regulatory peptides on human pancreatic cancer lines PANC-1 and MIA PaCa-2. Gastroenterology **98** (1990) 1666-1674

[21] J.F.R. Robertson *et al*, Effect of gastrointestinal hormones and synthetic analogues on the growth of pancreatic cancer. Int J Cancer **63** (1995) 69-75

[22] K. Detjen *et al*, Transfected cholecystokinin receptors mediate growth inhibitory effects on human pancreatic cancer cell lines. Gastroenterology **112** (1997) 952-959

Molecular Pathogenesis of Pancreatic Cancer
T.M. Gress (Ed.)
IOS Press, 2000

Application of array technology for expression profiling analyses of pancreatic cancer tissues and cells

C.Wenger*, F.Müller-Pillasch*, M.Buchholz, C.Wallrapp, V.Ellenrieder, G.Adler, T.M. Gress
Department of Internal Medicine I, Universitätsklinikum Ulm, 89081 Ulm, Germany

The development of new treatment modalities, diagnostic and preventive approaches for pancreatic cancer requires the understanding of the molecular mechanisms of the complex multistep process of tumourigenesis. At present mutations or alterations of gene expression have been described for a number of individual genes [1]. However, a much larger number of genes are warranted to be involved in primary and secondary processes responsible for the development of the phenotype of pancreatic cancer cells. Identification of these genes is essential as a basis for the development of new treatment or diagnostic modalities. Array-/chip-technology represents the ideal tool for a large scale analysis of complex genetic alterations in cancer and for the identification of new candidate genes of biomedical importance. In the recent years the major focus of our group has been to modify and adapt array-/chip-technology for the study of transcriptional alterations in pancreatic cancer tissues and cell lines. The present article summarizes a selection of our present and future strategies as well as some exemplary results obtained during the last years.

Use of array technology for expression profiling analyses of pancreatic cancer tissues

At the start of the project in 1991 gridded arrays of in-situ clones of gene libraries were used to study the complex alterations of gene expression occuring in pancreatic cancer cells, since DNA microarrays were not available at that time. We used gridded cDNA libraries from pancreatic cancer cell lines for differential hybridizations with labelled probes of the comple*te mRNA of pancreatic cancer and pancreatic control tissues [2]. These hybridizations allowed the detection of clones containing sequences abundantly expressed in the tissues used to generate the probe. Computerized subtraction analysis of hybridization results revealed that 4% of the total number of clones were selectively overexpressed in pancreatic carcinoma. A total of 410 cDNA clones (369 distinct clones) classified as preferentially expressed in pancreatic cancer were isolated from one cDNA library and characterized by Northern blot hybridizations, tag-sequencing and by screening nucleic acid or protein databases for sequence homologies. Northern blot hybridizations of 100 selected clones confirmed the hybridization pattern for approximately 90% of the clones. Tag-sequencing of the selected differentially expressed sequences identified novel genes (32,5 %) or homologues to EST-sequences with unknown function (26,3%). Homologies to known genes allowed to describe a pancreatic cancer-specific expression

* C.W. and F.M.P contributed equally to this manuscript and should both be considered first authors.

profile. The expression profile is summarized in figure 1. A large number of these differential genes were overexpressed in pancreatic cancer due to secondary alterations as for example increased energy metabolism or cellular turnover (structural and cytoskeletal genes, genes of the transcriptional and translational machinery). Knowledge of the genes involved in these mechanisms will help to understand the processes leading to increased proliferation and growth of cancer cells and may represent the basis for the development of treatment or diagnostic modalities.

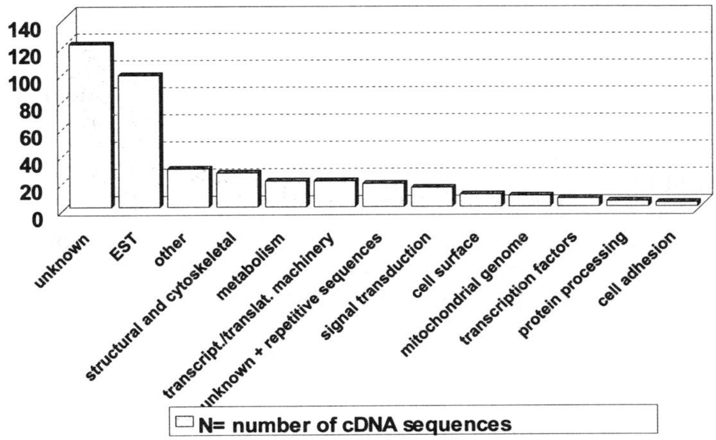

Figure 1
369 distinct ESTs classified as preferentially expressed in pancreatic cancer tissues were sorted into functional categories. The Y-axis shows the number of ESTs in each category (N°). [2]

One of our major interests besides the description of an expression profile of known genes was the identification of novel overexpressed genes suited as candidate disease genes. Since the tremendous improvements in array technology of the past years and the wider accessability it is no longer a technical challenge to generate expression profiles. However, the issue of selecting the right gene or genes e.g. as targets for pharmacological or diagnostic approaches is still not solved. Most of the expression profiling experiments done with the novel array technologies usually end with the generation of a large amount of expression data, which is difficult to handle and analyse. In the absence of a rational approach to the interpretation and exploitation of expression profiles the value of this data will be limited. For these reasons during the last years one of the major goals of our group was to develop strategies allowing to use expression profiles for the selection of genes of biomedical importance. Some of these strategies are described below.

Selection of new members of gene families with interesting biological functions

Initially we selected differentially expressed cDNA-sequences showing homologies to interesting genes or to sequence motifs of gene families of potential interest for pancreatic cancerogenesis. This led for example to the identification of a novel gene encoding a protein with four K-homologous (KH) domains, which was named *koc* (KH domain containing protein overexpressed in cancer. As the KH domain has been shown to be involved in the regulation of RNA synthesis and metabolism, *koc* may be involved in the regulation of transcriptional and/or posttranscriptional processes [3]. In the meantime we could show that this gene appears to be ubiquitously expressed at early stages of mouse and Xenopus embryonic development and thus represents a classical oncofetal [4]. Further interesting candidates were a gene encoding a novel putative tetraspan transmembrane protein highly homologous to the tumor associated antigen L6 (named *TM4SF5* for transmembrane 4 superfamily member 5) [5] and a gene encoding a novel putative transmembrane protein with two Kunitz-type serine protease inhibitor domains which was named *kop* (Kunitz domain containing protein overexpressed in pancreatic cancer). Being a member of the Kunitz-type serine protease inhibitor family, the *kop* gene may participate in tumor cell invasion and metastasis and in the development of the marked desmoplastic reaction typical for human pancreatic cancer tissues [6].

Use of array technology for the selection of candidate genes of biomedical importance

Usually only a fraction of the novel genes identified in an expression profiling approach will contain homologies to protein motifs allowing to draw functional conclusions. Thus, the approach described above will suffice for the selection of a small number of interesting candidates, but certainly does not represent a rational approach to the large amount of data generated in an expression profiling experiment. In our view one of the best ways to cope with the large number of possible candidate genes identified in an expression profiling apporach is the use of array-/chip-technology. It is our central strategy to use array-/chip-technology to accumulate further biological data for each individual gene selected in an expression profiling experiment.

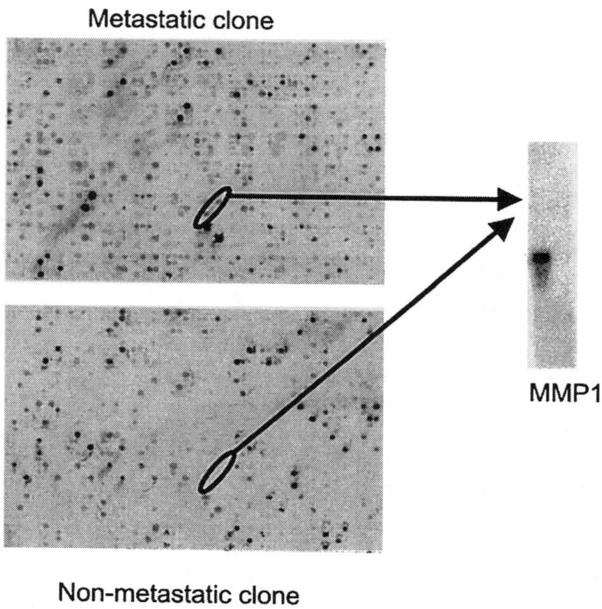

Figure 2

Hybridisation of an array of genes selected for being overexpressed in pancreatic cancer with the ^{33}P labelled mRNA of two pancreatic cancer cell lines differing in their metastatic potential. This hybridisation revealed a number of known and novel metastasis-associated genes as e.g. MMP1 (arrow). A Northern blot is shown confirming the differential expression of MMP1 in the metastatic clone.

As it is expensive and unwieldy to perform these sort of analyses with large gene arrays we usually prefer to generate smaller arrays/chips of all candidate genes identified in a large expression profiling approach. In the case of the first pancreatic cancer-specific expression profile described by our group [2] around 500 genes identified in this and further experiments were included in an array for further characterisation. These arrays contain all genes spotted in duplicate as in-situ colonies or ideally as PCR-products, as well as a number of control genes as e.g. housekeeping genes, vector genes and arabidopsis or yeast genes to precisely monitor further expression profiling hybridisations. This array is now used for hybridisations with the labelled mRNA of in-vitro or in-vivo model systems. These experiments allow us to identify genes associated with the major phenotypic characteristics of the respective in-vitro or in-vivo models. In this context we are e.g. using clones from one pancreatic cancer cell line differing in their metastatic potential to identify those genes on our array associated with the metastatic or invasive phenotype of pancreatic cancer cells (figure 2). Similar hybridisations are done to identify genes transcriptionally regulated by growth factors of major importance for the pathogenesis of pancreatic cancer as EGF or TGFβ [7, 8]. This is done by hybridising the labelled mRNA of pancreatic cancer cell lines treated or untreated with the respective growth factor onto our arrays. Alternatively cell lines stably transfected with constitutively active or dominant negative components of the downstream signalling cascades of the respective growth factors are used. Two types of hybridisation protocols can be used for these experiments. The first is used as standard in most expression profiling approaches and includes direct labelling of the mRNA directly either during or after reverse transcription with ^{33}P or fluorescence. This protocol allows to quantify the expression levels of all genes on the array in the respective mRNA used for hybridisation. This protocol may, however, miss differences on low expression levels and generate spurios results. Individual expression profiling experiments done with the same probe on the same array may differ considerably, so that a number of precautions should be taken. To solve the problem of sensitivity we presently prefer to use ^{33}P labelled rather than fluorescently labelled nucleotides. In general the sensitivity of radioactive probes is one log scale higher than of fluorescent probes. To exclude artifacts due to interexperimental variations each in-vitro experiment should at least be done in duplicate and each labelled probe from an in-vitro or in-vivo model should be hybridised at least three times on the same array. Alternatively, protocols can be used to enrich the mRNA for differential genes prior to labelling and hybridisation. This can be done by using protocols as e.g. subtractive supression hybridisation (SSH) [9] or representational difference analysis (RDA) [10]. We have optimized the cDNA-RDA approach to generate enriched probes for array hybridisations with great success. CDNA-RDA represents an iterative process of subtractive hybridization and selective PCR-amplification allowing to select differentially expressed genes with a highly reproducible specificity. RDA was originally deviced to clone differences between complex genomes [11]. The RDA protocol was later adapted for the use with cDNA to study differential gene expression between two mRNA populations, the so-called “tester” (containing the sequences to be enriched) and “driver” (containing the sequences to be subtracted) [12]. The standard cDNA RDA-protocol is ideally suited to rapidly reduce the number of candidate genes in a highly specific manner, thus allowing to focus on a small number of differential genes [10]. We decided to test the use of RDA-products as probes for array hybridisations [13] to provide a straight-forward and reliable protocol which eliminates the problems usually encountered during standard expression profiling hybridisations with the labelled mRNA or cDNA. The difference products (DP) of representational difference analyses (RDA) were used as hybridization probes on cDNA arrays. The effectivity of RDA-products obtained with increasing driver/tester ratios (DP 1 = 100 : 1, DP 2 = 800 : 1, DP 3 = 400 000 : 1) to isolate differentially expressed genes in pancreatic cancer was tested. In this approach the hybridization with the DP2 product obtained after the second round of RDA at a driver/tester ratio of 800:1 represented the best compromise between yield and specificity. The yield was comparable to standard differential hybridizations, whereas the fraction of genes selectively overexpressed in pancreatic cancer tissues was higher. In summary, this new technique is well suited for the isolation of genes differentially expressed in cancer tissues combining the advantages of gridded arrays and cDNA representational difference analysis. This technique is an attractive alternative to conventional expression profiling hybridisations with gridded arrays as it provides a higher specificity (in general it is sufficient to hybridise each enriched probe once) and it produces hybridization results allowing a reliable and convenient data analysis with an automated system or even by eye.

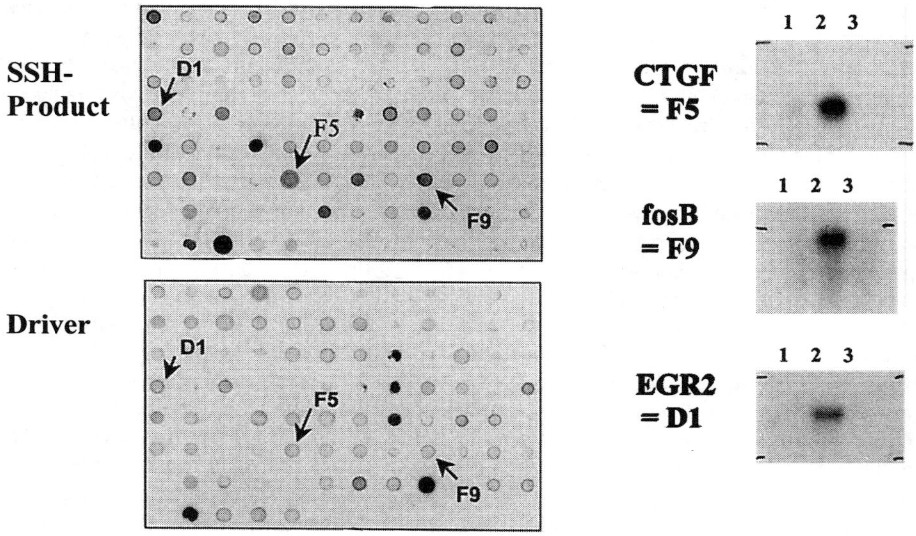

Figure 3

A small array with selected genes was hybridised with ^{33}P labelled driver and the SSH product obtained in an experiment designed to isolate early reponse genes of EGF in pancreatic cancer cell lines. mRNA from the cell line PANC-1 treated for 1h with 50 ng/ml EGF was used as *tester* and mRNA from PANC-1 cells treated with meium only was used as *driver* for a standard subtractive suppression hybridisation approach. Hybridisations with arrays identified several early response genes of EGF and the confirmatory Northern blot hybridisations for a selection of these genes are shown in the figure. Each lane on the Northern blots contains 20 μg of total RNA from PANC-1 cells after 0h (1), 1h (2) and 4h (3) of treatment with EGF.

In this context one approach designed to isolate target genes of EGF/TGFα led to the identification of connective tissue growth factor (CTGF) as interesting gene for the pathogenesis of pancreatic cancer. *CTGF* is an immediate early growth responsive gene that has been shown to be a downstream mediator of TGFβ actions in fibroblasts and vascular endothelial cells. In the present study using array technology and subtractive suppression hybridisation (SSH) h*CTGF* was isolated as immediate early target gene of EGF/TGFα in human pancreatic cancer cells [8]. *CTGF* transcripts were found in 13/15 pancreatic cancer cell lines incubated with 10% serum. In 3/7 pancreatic cancer cell lines EGF/TGFα induced a significant rise of *CTGF* transcript levels peaking 1-2 h after the start of treatment. TGFβ increased *CTGF* transcript levels in 2/7 pancreatic cancer cell lines after 4 h of treatment and this elevation was sustained after 24 h. Only treatment with TGFβ was accompanied by a parallel induction of *collagen type I* transcription. 15/19 human pancreatic cancer tissues were shown to overexpress high levels of *CTGF* transcripts. *CTGF* transcript levels in pancreatic cancer tissues and nude mouse xenograft tumors showed a good correlation to the degree of fibrosis. *In situ* hybridization and nude mouse experiments revealed that in pancreatic cancer tissues, fibroblasts are the predominant site of *CTGF* transcription, whereas the tumor cells appeared to contribute to a lesser extent. CTGF may thus be of paramount importance for the development of the characteristic desmoplastic reaction in pancreatic cancer tissues.

Summary and conclusion

In this article we have reviewed experiences from our group showing that the use of array technology can be invaluabale to identify new targets of biomedical importance for cancer research. Since the advances of the last years have made this technology widely accessible it will become a standard tool in many laboratories. However, many issues will have to be solved to make maximal benefit of this technology. Issues as sensitivity, reproducibility, reliability as well as the rational bioinformatic and biological evaluation of expression profiling data are of major importance. This article summarizes some of the approaches we have employed to address these issues, which may be helpful for future array experiments.

Acknowledgements

This work was supported in part by grants from the European Union (BMH4-CT98-3085) and the Deutsche Forschungsgemeinschaft (SFB518, Projects B1 and C1) to TMG.

Literature

[1] S.E. Kern, Advances from genetic clues in pancreatic cancer. Curr Opin Oncol **10** (1998) 74-80.

[2] T.M. Gress *et al*, A pancreatic cancer-specific expression profile. Oncogene **13** (1996) 1819-1830.

[3] F. Mueller Pillasch *et al*, Cloning of a gene highly overexpressed in cancer coding for a novel KH-domain containing protein. Oncogene **14** (1997) 2729-2733.

[4] F.Müller-Pillasch *et al*, Expression of the highly conserved RNA-binding protein koc in embryogenesis. MOD **88** (1999) 95-99.

[5] F.Muller Pillasch *et al*, Identification of a new tumour-associated antigen TM4SF5 and its expression in human cancer. Gene **208** (1998) 25-30

[6] F. Muller Pillasch *et al*, Cloning of a new Kunitz-type protease inhibitor with a putative transmembrane domain overexpressed in pancreatic cancer. Biochim Biophys Acta **1395** (1998) 88-95.

[7] M.M.Geng *et al*, Use of representational difference analysis to study the effect of TGFβ on the expression profile of a pancreatic cancer cell line. Genes Chromosom. Cancer **26** (1999) 70-79.

[8] C.Wenger *et al*, Expression and Differential Regulation of *Connective Tissue Growth Factor* in Pancreatic Cancer Cells. Oncogene **18** (1999) 1073-1080.

[9] L. Diatchenko *et al*, Suppression subtractive hybridization: a method for generating differentially regulated or tissue-specific cDNA probes and libraries. Proc Natl Acad Sci USA **93** (1996) 6025-6030.

[10] T.M.Gress et al, Identification of genes with specific expression in pancreatic cancer by cDNA representational difference analysis. Genes Chromosomes Cancer **19** (1997) 97-103

[11] N. Lisitsyn *et al*, Cloning the differences between two complex genomes. Science 259 (1993) 946-951.

[12] M. Hubank and D.G. Schatz, Identifying differences in mRNA expression by representational difference analysis of cDNA. Nucleic Acids Res **22** (1994) 5640-5648.

[13] M.M. Geng *et a*l, Isolation of differentially expressed genes by combining representational difference analysis (RDA) and cDNA library arrays. BioTechniques **25/3** (1998) 434-438.

Molecular Pathogenesis of Pancreatic Cancer
T.M. Gress (Ed.)
IOS Press, 2000

The bHLH transcription factor p48 in exocrine pancreas differentiation *in vitro*

Teresa Adell, Anouchka Skoudy, Alicia Gómez-Cuadrado,
Teresa Palomero, and Francisco X. Real
Unitat de Biologia Cel.lular i Molecular, Institut Municipal d'Investigació Mèdica, Universitat Pompeu Fabra; Carrer del Dr. Aiguader, 80, E-08003 Barcelona, Spain

Pancreatic acinar cells display phenotypic plasticity and can switch to a ductal phenotype in vitro. Similarly, a switch from acinar to ductal phenotype can occur in chronic pancreatitis and pancreatic cancer. We have hypothesized that acinar-ductal conversion results from changes in the expression of transcription factors involved in exocrine differentiation. The PTF1 transcriptional complex, involved in the regulation of expression of acinar-specific genes, is a candidate. PTF1 is constituted by two ubiquitous bHLH proteins, p75 and p64, and a tissue-specific bHLH factor, p48. In normal exocrine pancreas cultures, down-regulation of acinar gene expression occurs already at 24 h of culture and is associated with a down-regulation of p48 but not of the other PTF1 components. To determine if reexpression of p48 is able to activate acinar gene expression, normal pancreas cultures were transfected with the rat p48 cDNA. p48 transfection did not activate acinar genes in normal exocrine cultures or in ductal-type pancreas cancer cells; by contrast, p48 transfection upregulated PTF1 activity in AR42J rat pancreas cancer cells. HNF-3β and PDX-1 have also been shown to contribute to acinar gene expression and both of them were present in normal pancreas cultures displaying a ductal phenotype. Our findings suggest that: 1) p48 may play a role in pancreatic disease and 2) normal pancreatic cultures display features reminiscent of pancreatic stem cells.

1. INTRODUCTION

Acinar cell-specific genes have been extensively used as models to study the regulation of gene expression [reviewed in 1]. Transcripts for pancreatic amylase, elastase, trypsinogen, and chymotrypsinogen, among others, are almost exclusively detected, using highly sensitive assays, in pancreatic acinar cells. Sequences 5' to the transcription initiation site of genes encoding these enzymes display significant homology and bind to a pancreas-specific transcriptional complex designated PTF1 [1]. PTF1 is a hetero-oligomeric complex composed by two non-pancreas specific subunits, designated p75 and p64, and the pancreas-specific component p48 [2,3]. These three proteins belong to the basic helix-loop-helix (bHLH) family of transcriptional regulators. p75 is a product of the E12/E47 gene whereas p64 is a product of REB (HEB in humans) [4]. By contrast, p48 belongs to the class B bHLH proteins and shares homology in the HLH region with twist and myoD [3]. p64 and p48 form a heterodimer and bind directly to DNA whereas p75 is involved in nuclear transport of the complex and does not bind DNA [5,6]. p48 contacts the CANNTG sequence in the enhancer region of genes coding for acinar enzymes and it is essential for their expression [5]: antisense-induced down-regulation of p48 is associated with the inactivation of the exocrine programme in rat AR42J tumor cells [3]. Genetic inactivation of the p48 gene in mice leads to an apancreatic phenotype characterized by the complete lack of exocrine tissue and the presence of a reduced number of isolated endocrine cells in the spleen [7]. Despite the crucial role of p48 in exocrine pancreas development and function, other transcription factors, such as HNF-3β and PDX-1, are also required for efficient expression of acinar genes [8,9]. HNF-3β is activated in the endoderm and PDX-1 is expressed in the endoderm at the level of the prospective pancreatic epithelium and is essential for pancreatic development [10].

Unlike the extensive knowledge about the genetic elements and transcriptional regulatory complexes involved in acinar gene expression, very limited information is available on the regulation of expression of duct cell markers [11]. Transgenes have been reproducibly and selectively targeted to pancreatic acinar cells [1,12]; by contrast, they have been rarely targeted to ductal cells [13]. Furthermore, little is known regarding the transcription factors that may be involved in the activation of a ductal differentiation programme in the pancreas.

Acinar, ductal, and islet cells are ontogenetically related. After the emergence of the dorsal and ventral buds during pancreatic development, glucagon expression is detected, branching morphogenesis takes place, and insulin and acinar cell-specific products are detected later [reviewed in 14]. Several other observations support a close lineage relationship between acinar and ductal pancreatic cells. Among them are the acinar-ductal phenotypical switch reported in tumors of transgenic mice in which c-myc is targeted to acinar cells using the elastase promoter [15] and in rat tumors induced by azaserine [16,17]. Furthermore, such a switch is not restricted to transformed cells. We and others have shown that when the exocrine fraction of human pancreas, containing 90% acinar cells, is placed in culture, acinar cell markers are rapidly down-regulated as ductal markers are up-regulated [18,19]. After 10 days of culture, normal human exocrine cells had not only acquired a ductal phenotype but ductal functional properties, such as response to secretin, as well [18]. The limited proliferative activity of these cells and the lack of extensive cell death in vitro point to an acinar-to-ductal conversion, or transdifferentiation, rather than to the selective outgrowth of ductal cells [18,19]. This phenotypical switch is of considerable interest because it is reminiscent of that observed in ductular complexes associated with chronic pancreatitis both in man and in experimental models in rodents [11,20].

The phenotypical changes described above have prompted us to examine the molecular mechanisms involved in the acinar-ductal conversion as they might shed light on the mechanisms involved in pancreatic pathology, such as chronic pancreatitis and pancreatic cancer. The hypothesis that the PTF1 complex, HNF-3β, and/or PDX-1 might play a role in such processes is adressed in this work.

2. RESULTS

2.1. The acinar-ductal phenotypical switch in normal exocrine pancreas cultures. The kinetics of the phenotypical switch that occurs during the culture of normal exocrine pancreas cells was analyzed by northern blotting using probes for acinar markers (lipase and chymotrypsinogen) and ductal markers [cystic fibrosis transmembrane regulator (CFTR) and cytokeratin 7 (K7)]. K8 was also analyzed because it is expressed in both acinar and ductal cells. As shown in Figure 1, lipase and chymotrypsinogen transcript levels were high in cultured cells at day 1, low on day 3, and almost undetectable by day 6. By contrast, the levels of CFTR and K7 transcripts were undetectable at days 1 and 3 and were up-regulated by day 6 and 10. Similarly, immunocytochemical assays on cells cultured for ≥6 days showed that amylase was undetectable; by contrast, 100% of cells were found to express K7 and K18 [18]. These findings indicate that the extinction of the acinar differentiation programme is an early event.

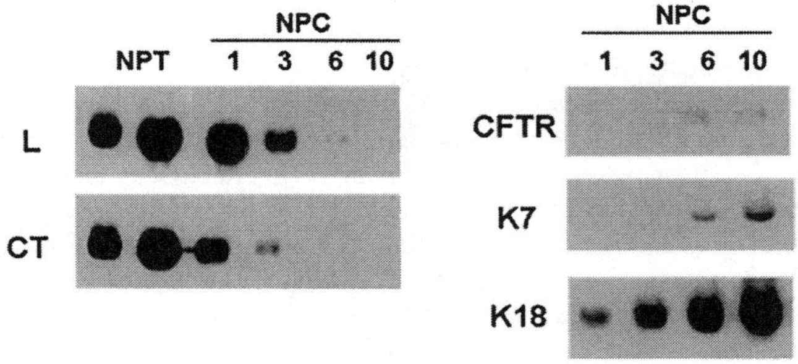

Figure 1. Acinar cells undergo <u>in vitro</u> a phenotypical switch characterized by the loss of acinar cell markers and the up-regulation of ductal cell markers. Normal human exocrine pancreas cultures (NPC) were established as previously described [18]. Total RNA isolated using guanidium isothiocyanate from cultured cells and normal pancreas tissue (NPT) was fractionated by agarose gel electrophoresis, transferred to nylon filters, and hybridized with probes for acinar (L, lipase; CT, chymotrypsinogen) and ductal cell markers (CFTR; K7). Cytokeratin 8 (K8) was detected in both types of cells but levels were higher in ductal cells.

2.2. Expression of PTF1 complex components in the course of the acinar-ductal phenotypical switch. To determine if changes in the levels of expression of p48 may be involved in the loss of acinar features and the acquisition of ductal characteristics, RT-PCR (Figure 2A) and western blotting (Figure 2B) were performed. Using a nested PCR, p48 mRNA was detected in samples from pancreas tissue but not from cultured cells after day 1. Anti-p48 antibodies were reactive with normal rat and human pancreas tissues and with the isolated exocrine pancreas fraction (day 0), though the levels were lower than in tissue. At day 1, p48 levels had clearly decreased and the protein was no longer detectable at later timepoints. Amylase followed the variation of p48 levels in cultured cells though it was detectable up to day 4, likely as a result of the very high levels present in the exocrine pancreas. Similar results were obtained using immunocytochemical techniques (Figure 2C).

To examine if the other components of the PTF1 complex are similarly down-regulated, RT-PCR assays were performed using primers specific of the E12 and E47 transcripts of the E2A gene and HEB [17]. As shown in Figure 3, E2A and HEB transcripts were consistently detected through the culture. Anti-E2A antibodies recognized a 70 kDa protein in cultured cells; anti-HEB antibodies recognized proteins of 58 kDa, 68 kDa, and 84 kDa the identity of which remains to be established (data not shown).

To confirm that the PTF1 complex is lost upon culture of normal pancreas, electrophoretic mobility shift assays were performed using ^{32}P-labeled oligonucleotides corresponding to the sequences of the A element of the human elastase-3 enhancer. A complex that was specifically inhibited by the same unlabeled oligonucleotide, but not by

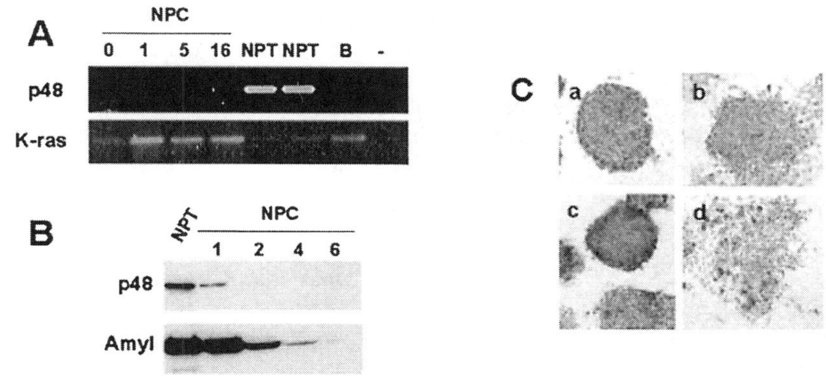

Figure 2. p48 in normal pancreas tissue (NPT) and cultured cells (NPC). *Panel A*: Transcripts coding for p48 were analyzed by RT-PCR as described elsewhere [17]. K-ras transcripts were amplified as control of cDNA quality. *Panel B*: p48 and amylase levels in normal pancreas tissue and cultured cells detected by western blotting. The production and specificity of anti-p48 antibodies have been reported elsewhere [17]; anti-amylase antibodies were purchased from Sigma Chemical Co. (St. Louis, MO). *Panel C*: Immunocytochemical detection of p48 and amylase in normal pancreas cultures at day 1 (a, c) or day 4 (b, d) of culture. Anti-p48 (a, b); anti-amylase (c, d). NPC, normal exocrine pancreas cultures; NPT, normal pancreas tissue; B, gallbladder; -, H_2O control.

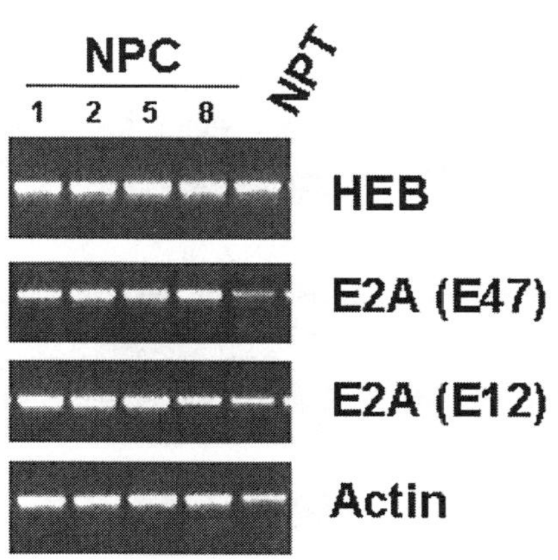

Figure 3. RT-PCR analysis of E2A (E47 and E12) and HEB transcripts in normal human pancreas tissue (NPT) and cultured cells (NPC). Actin is shown as a control for cDNA amplification. Primers and PCR conditions were as reported elsewhere [17].

an irrelevant oligonucleotide, was detected using nuclear extracts from normal pancreas tissue and the exocrine pancreas fraction at day 0, but not with extracts from cells cultured at day 6 nor from non-pancreatic cells. Formation of this complex was inhibited by anti-p48 antibodies but not by preimmune rabbit serum (data not shown).

Altogether, these results indicate that in normal exocrine pancreas cultures the PTF1 complex is rapidly lost and this is associated with the down-regulation of p48.

2.3. Activation of acinar gene expression by p48 in transient transfection assays. To determine if p48 is able to activate the acinar differentiation programme in pancreatic cells displaying a ductal phenotype, normal pancreatic cultures were transiently transfected with the rat p48 cDNA and amylase was analyzed in cell lysates and culture medium. Despite the low efficiecy of transfection of normal pancreatic cells, p48 was detected by western blotting in cultures transfected with p48 cDNA but not in those transfected with control vector. Amylase was undetectable in both cultures (Figure 4). While we cannot rule that these results are due to the fact that the rat p48 cDNA was transfected into human cells, other transcription factors of the bHLH family, such as MyoD, are active in these type of assays across species barriers.

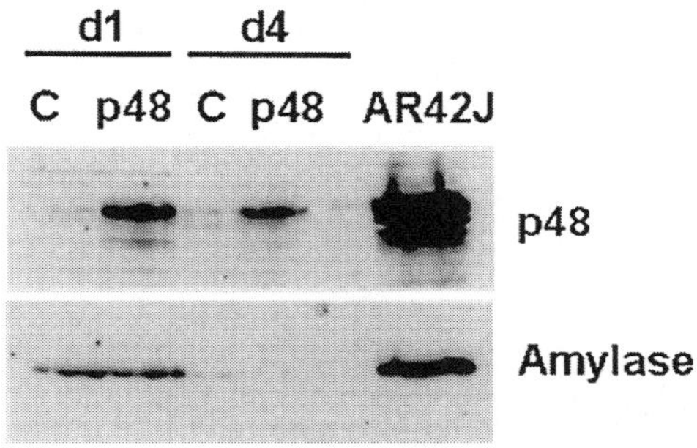

Figure 4. Transient transfection of p48 cDNA into normal exocrine pancreatic cultured cells at days 1 and 4. Normal human exocrine pancreas cells were seeded on Petri dishes and transfected at days 1 or 4 either with empty vector (pcDNA.3, C) or with the same vector containing the full length rat p48 cDNA (pCDNA3.p48) using Lipofectamine (Lipofectamine Plus Reagent, Gibco), following manufacturer's instructions. Cell lysates were prepared 48 h after transfection and used for detection of p48 and amylase by western blotting. AR42J cell lysates shown as control.

2.4. Expression of HNF-3β and PDX-1 in the course of the acinar-ductal phenotypical switch. HNF-3β and PDX-1 are also involved in the regulation of the expression of acinar genes [8,9]. Western blotting analysis using nuclear extracts from normal exocrine cultures showed detectable levels of HNF-3β throughout the culture period. As reported by other authors, anti-PDX-1 antibodies detected two components at all times of culture; their precise significance has not yet been established. The expression of HNF-3β and PDX-1 in these cells is reminiscent of the phenotype of pancreatic precursors found at early stages of pancreatic development [14].

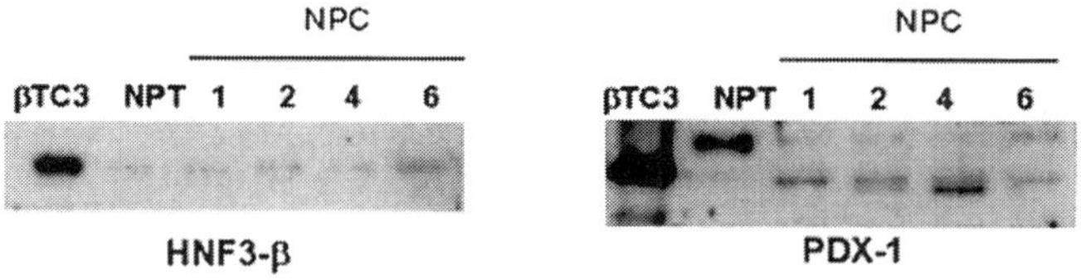

Figure 5. Expression of HNF-3β and PDX-1 in pancreatic cells using western blotting. humanpancreas tissue; NPC, normal exocrine pancreas cultures. βTC3 cells are shown as positive control.

2.5. PTF-1 component expression in rat pancreas cancer cells with a ductal phenotype obtained by in vitro culture of azaserine-induced acinar tumor cells. The azaserine-induced rat pancreatic tumors display an acinar phenotype that is lost upon in vitro culture. p48 mRNA and protein were detected in tissue from acinar tumors. By contrast, cultured cells derived from these tumors displaying a ductal phenotype lacked expression of p48 while retaining expression of transcripts corresponding to the other two subunits of the PTF-1 complex [17]. Transfection of rat p48 cDNA into cells with a ductal phenotype did not result in the activation of the exocrine differentiation programme [17].

3. DISCUSSION

Our studies show that p48 expression is absent from normal and neoplastic cells undergoing an acinar-ductal phenotypical switch, while expression of the remaining components of the PTF-1 complex is retained, at least at the mRNA level. In addition, reexpression of p48 by transfection is not accompanied by the reactivation of the acinar phenotype [this work and reference 17]. Altogether, these data support the notion that other molecular changes take place in the course of this phenotypical switch that can not be overcome by p48 reexpression; changes in the expression of Ids [21], negative regulators of the bHLH family such as Twist [22], or in the structure of chromatin, for example through modification of histone acetylation [23], might contribute to these effects.

In addition to the absence of p48 mRNA, recent work from our laboratory has shown that the subcellular distribution of p48 may also contribute to its functional inactivation: in AR42J cells, p48 was mainly targeted to the nucleus whereas in human (RWP1) and rat (DSL6) pancreas cancer cells, it accumulated in the cytoplasm despite the expression of p75 mRNA [17]. More work is necessary to establish the molecular mechanisms involved in the observed cytoplasmic accumulation.

Little is known about the regulation of p48 expression. Up to 10 kb upstream of the transcription initiation site have been analyzed functionally by transfection but no clear-cut evidence of pancreas-specific sequences has thus far been obtained [24], suggesting that regulatory elements are far from the coding sequences and/or the participation of a complex code of transcriptional regulators. Transgenic mice in which a dominant negative Notch3 mutant protein is expressed under the control of the Pdx-1 promoter in the embryonic pancreatic epithelium display small pancreatic buds with reduced expression of Hes and p48 transcripts, suggesting that the Notch pathway is involved in proliferation, morphogenesis, and exocrine differentiation in the pancreas [25].

The phenotype of the cultured cells described here, including the expression of HNF-3β and PDX-1, is reminiscent of the phenotype of pancreatic embryonic precursors [14] as these transcription factors are expressed in the fetal epithelium and subsequently down-regulated in normal adult ductal cells. Therefore, it may be possible to genetically manipulate these cells, so that the exocrine and/or endocrine differentiation programmes are activated, and use them for transplantation.

The findings described above are of relevance to human pancreatic disease: an acinar-ductal conversion similar to that observed in the cultured cells takes place in chronic pancreatitis and in the course of neoplastic transformation of the pancreatic epithelium, at least in experimental animals [26,27]. Recent work has shown that the Pdx-1-expressing pool of cells is amplified in chronic pancreatitis lesions in mice in which the TGF-α gene is overexpressed under the control of the metallothionin promoter [20]. A better understanding of the in vitro phenotypical switch may shed light on the molecular pathways involved in disease conditions and lead to novel therapeutic strategies.

Acknowledgments

This work was supported in part by grants from Comisión Interministerial de Ciencia y Tecnología (SAF94-0971), Dirección General de Enseñanza Superior e Investigación Científica (PM97-0077), Generalitat de Catalunya (SGR-00433), and Biomed Programme (BMH4-CT98-3085). T.A. and A.S. were recipients of grants from CIRIT (Generalitat de Catalunya). We thank D.S. Longnecker, A. Scarpa, C. Figarella, E. Fuchs, and X. Estivill for providing cells and probes, and O. Hagenbüchle for providing the rat p48 cDNA and for many valuable discussions.

References

[1] R. J. MacDonald and G. H. Swift. Analysis of transcriptional regulatory regions in vivo. Int. J. Dev. Biol. **42** (1998) 42983-94.

[2] M. Cockell *et al.*, Identification of a cell-specific DNA-binding activity that interacts with a transcriptional activator of genes expressed in the acinar pancreas. Mol. Cell. Biol. **9** (1989) 2464-2476.

[3] A. Krapp *et al.*, The p48 DNA-binding subunit of transcription factor PTF1 is a new exocrine pancreas-specific basic helix-loop-helix protein. EMBO J. **15** (1996) 4317-4329.

[4] O. Hagenbüchle *et al.*, The bHLH protein p48, a DNA-binding subunit of PTF1, acts as a morphogen during pancreas development. Exp. Clin. Endocrinol. Diabetes **105** (1997) 4(A9).

[5] E. Roux *et al.*, The cell-specific transcription factor PTF1 contains two different subunits that interact with the DNA. Genes Dev. **3** (1989) 1613-1624.

[6] L. Sommer *et al.*, Nuclear targeting of the transcription factor PTF1 is mediated by a protein subunit that does not bind to the PTF1 cognate sequence. Cell **67** (1991) 987-994.

[7] A. Krapp *et al.*, The bHLH protein PTF1-p48 is essential for the formation of the exocrine and the correct spatial organization of the endocrine pancreas. Genes Dev. **12** (1998) 3752-3763.

[8] M. Cockell *et al.*, Binding sites for hepatocyte nuclear factor 3β or 3γ and pancreas transcription factor 1 are required for efficient expression of the gene encoding pancreatic α-amylase. Mol. Cell. Biol. **15** (1995) 1933-1941.

[9] G. H. Swift *et al.*, An endocrine-exocrine switch in the activity of the pancreatic homeodomain protein PDX1 through formation of a trimeric complex with PBX1b and MRG1 (MEIS2). Mol. Cell. Biol. **18** (1998) 5109-5120.
[10] J. Jonsson *et al.*, Insulin-promoter-factor 1 is required for pancreas development in mice. Nature **371** (1994) 606-609.
[11] F. X. Real, The cell biology of pancreatic cancer. In: J. Neoptolemos, N.R. Lemoine (eds), Pancreatic Cancer, Blackwell Science Press, Oxford, 1995, pp. 3-17.
[12] S. D. Rose *et al.*, A single element of the elastase I enhancer is sufficient to direct transcription selectively to the pancreas and gut. Mol. Cell. Biol. **14** (1994) 2048-2057.
[13] T. L. Jetton *et al.*, Targeted oncogenesis of hormone-negative islet progenitor cells. Proc. Natl. Acad. Sci. USA **95** (1998) 8654-8659.
[14] H. Edlund, Pancreas: how to get there from the gut. Curr. Opin. Cell Biol. **11** (1999) 663-668.
[15] E. P. Sandgren *et al.*, Pancreatic tumor pathogenesis reflects the causative genetic lesion. Proc. Natl. Acad. Sci. USA **88** (1991) 93-97.
[16] O. S. Pettengill *et al.*, Derivation of ductlike cell lines from transplantable acinar cell carcinoma of the rat pancreas. Am. J. Pathol. **143** (1993) 292-303.
[17] T. Adell *et al.*, Role of the basic helix-loop-helix transcription factor p48 in the differentiation phenotype of exocrine pancreas cancer cells. Cell Growth Diff. (2000) in press.
[18] M. R. Vilá *et al.*, Normal human pancreas cultures display functional ductal characteristics. Lab. Invest. **71** (1994) 423-431.
[19] P. A. Hall and N. Lemoine. Rapid acinar to ductal transdifferentiation in cultured human exocrine pancreas. J. Pathol. **166** (1992) 97-103.
[20] S. Y. Song *et al.*, Expansion of Pdx1-expressing pancreatic epithelium and islet neogenesis in transgenic mice overexpressing transforming growth factor α. Gastroenterology **117** (1999) 1416-1426.
[21] J. D. Norton *et al.*, *Id* helix-loop-helix proteins in cell growth and differentiation. Trends Cell Biol. **8** (1998) 58-65.
[22] D. B. Spicer *et al.*, Inhibition of myogenic bHLH and MEF-2 transcription factors by the bHLH protein twist. Science **272** (1996) 1476-1480.
[23] B. D. Strahl and C. D. Allis, The language of covalent histone modifications. Nature **403** (2000) 41-45.
[24] M. Knöffler *et al.*, Constitutive expression of the gene for the cell-specific p48 DNA-binding subunit of pancreas transcription factor 1 in cultured cells is under control of binding sites for transcription factors Sp1 and alpha Cbf. J. Biol. Chem. **271** (1996) 21993-22002.
[25] A. Apelqvist *et al.*, Notch signalling controls pancreatic cell differentiation. Nature **400** (1999) 877-881.
[26] D. M. Scarpelli *et al.*, Are acinar cells involved in the pathogenesis of ductal adenocarcinoma of the pancreas? Cancer Cells **3** (1991) 275-277.
[27] M. Wagner *et al.*, Malignant transformation of duct-like cells originating from acini in transforming growth factor α transgenic mice. Gastroenterology **115** (1998) 1254-1262.

Molecular Pathogenesis of Pancreatic Cancer
T.M. Gress (Ed.)
IOS Press, 2000

Chips, arrays and other hybridisation based techniques for genome and transcriptome characterisation

Marcus Frohme, Nicole Hauser, Marcel Scheideler,
Frank Diehl, Markus Beier, Simone Würtz and Jörg D. Hoheisel

Department of Functional Genome Analysis,
Deutsches Krebsforschungszentrum, Heidelberg, Germany

The characterisation of complete genomic sequences and the transcriptional activity of their coding portions is a current focus in the quest for a broad understanding of the functioning and the regulative factors of the information encoded in the genes. Functional analysis actually extends already beyond comprehensive studies at only the level of DNA and RNA, termed genome and transcriptome research, respectively, to global investigations of the cellular content of proteins and metabolites and studies on their interaction, scientific fields nowadays associated with the terms proteome and metabolome analysis. While proteins and metabolites are not easily accessible to scientific scrutiny, however, nucleic acids are comparatively uncomplicated with regard to handling - one reason for this being their relatively simple structural basis with only a restricted degree of variation possible - and much more amicable to high throughput analyses and means of automatisation. One of the major methodologies used to such ends is hybridisation of nucleic acid to a matrix of potentially homologous probe molecules. These probes can be free in solution or attached to solid support, which can be either of a more flexible, porous kind like a membrane or filter made of nylon or nitrocellulose or a flat and rigid structure such as glass slides, polypropylene sheets or silicon wafers. Particularly the arrays on rigid support media are often referred to as DNA-chips. Because of the intrinsic parallelism, analysis is economised. Therefore, investigation of large numbers of possible targets is made practical.

One of the major goals of functional genome analyses is the detection of differentially expressed genes, thus bringing their mere existence in a functional context, from which the actual activity of the related protein and the regulation of the expression could be derived. To this end, several methods have been developed in the last decade. A highly selective one is representational difference analysis, which requires no prior knowledge about the genome. In well-known systems, arrayed cDNA-clones or PCR-products form the technical basis for the generation of transcriptional profiles that report globally on gene activity. Functional analysis also looks for genomic variation, namely the detection of mutations, especially if of medical interest. Simultaneous to the experimental approaches, new hardware did evolve and algorithms for data evaluation, management and sensible interpretation are being developed in the area of bioinformatics. All those types of hybridisation-mediated analysis are discussed below based on examples elaborated in our group.

cDNA-RDA for the detection of new cancer genes

Representational difference analysis (RDA; Fig. 1) - described in more detail elsewhere in this book - is suitable to detect alterations on both the genomic [1] and transcriptional level [2]. In the latter case, the main objective is an identification of genes, which are differentially transcribed in two samples. Starting material might be tumour tissue, for example, compared to a related normal sample. Complex cDNAs, representing the expression state of both tissues, are cut, ligated with adapters and PCR-amplified, resulting in mixtures of PCR-fragments that should be representative of the respective starting material. These "representations" serve as tester and driver in a subsequent iterative process of selective amplification of fragments more frequent in the tester fraction (Fig. 1).

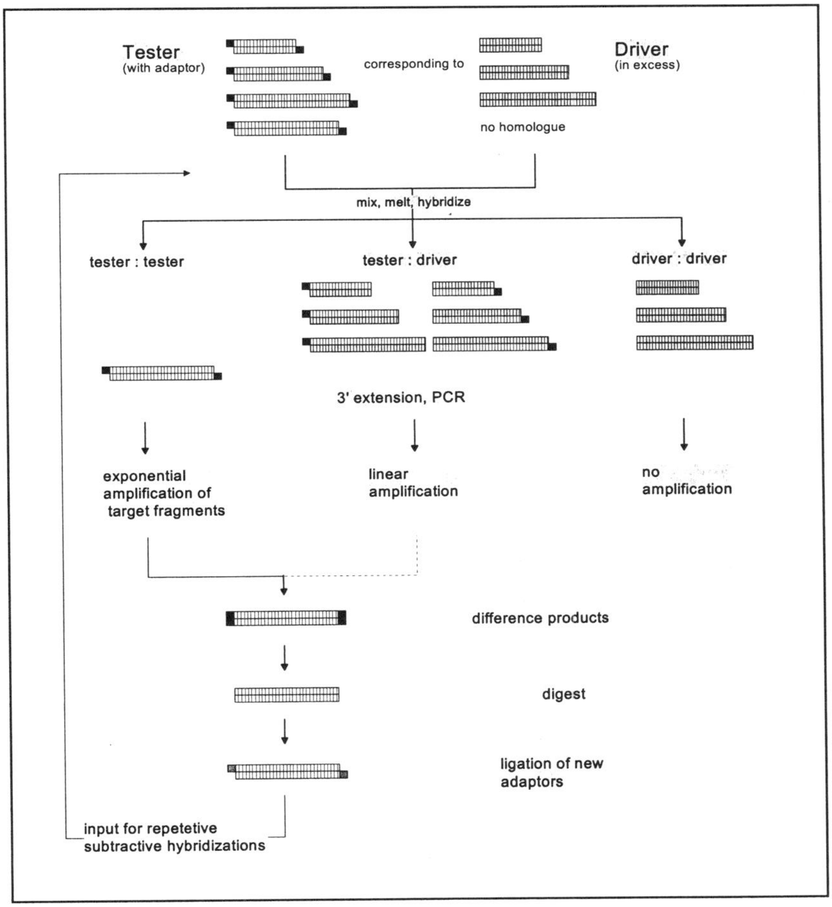

Fig. 1: Principle of RDA (without the generation of the representations). Tester and driver are mixed and denatured. The driver excess competes out homologous tester fragments in a hybridisation governed by a subtractive and a kinetic component. Only molecules formed of strands that both originate from the tester are exponentially amplifiable in subsequent PCR.

These difference products are eventually cloned for further analysis. Fixation of the fragments on suitable supports like membranes (Fig. 2) or glass (Fig. 5) creates arrays, which serve for the validation of the experiment [3]. Labelled samples made from the two original RNA preparations or the related cDNA are hybridised to such an array in an experiment sometimes also called reverse Northern blot. The comparison of the signals obtained in both experiments checks the accuracy of the experimental process. Real and potential false positives are immediately identified, if present in the original RNA/cDNA-sample frequently enough in order to produce directly sufficient signal. Usually, this simple experiment is enough for an overall confirmation of the experiment's success. For individual clones, however, further proof by other means might be necessary, such as *in situ* hybridisation or PCR, if their signal intensity is too weak or the degree of quantification insufficient. Technically, RDA only selects for an increase in molecule numbers, hence up-regulation. However, if either representation of a pair is used both as a tester and a driver in separate, reverse experiments, up-regulation and down-regulation of genes will be found.

The application of RDA is particularly of interest in biological systems, of which not all genes have yet been identified by sequencing (as still is the case in human, although this will change very soon). Another major advantage is the enormous sensitivity and selectivity, which in addition can be adapted by variation of the driver/tester ratios and the kinetic parameters.

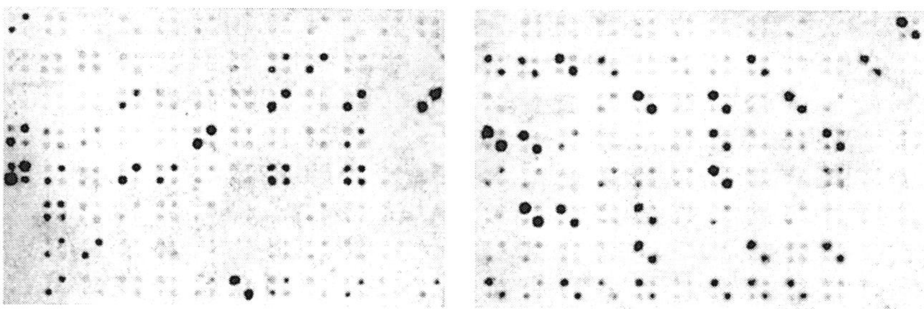

Fig. 2: Confirmation of RDA results. Amplified difference products of an experiment with larynx tumour material as tester and RNA from normal tissue as driver were spotted in duplicate in a right-diagonal orientation (.˙); the products of the reverse experiment (healthy tissue as tester) were spotted in a left-diagonal orientation (˙.) on the same nylon membrane. Hybridisation with radioactively labelled cDNA of the tumour tissue (left panel) and the healthy tissue (right panel) confirmed in most cases the up- or down-regulation of the genes in the tumour.

Transcriptional profiling and data management

Another approach toward the identification of differentially transcribed genes is the array-based analysis of many genes in parallel [4]. Prerequisite is the availability of sequences either in form of genomic sequence, from which coding portions can be defined, or cDNA. The latter should be of low redundancy and ideally already sequenced. Gene-specific or vector primers are used for the amplification of the sequences. The products are arrayed on membranes or chips, usually by robotic devices in order to achieve high densities. Targets of complex cDNA preparations originating from different tissues or vary in other experimental conditions are then hybridised. For many spots on the support, the signal intensities will not change between various experiments. Different signal intensities correspond to different concentrations of the particular RNA molecule in the sample (Fig. 3).

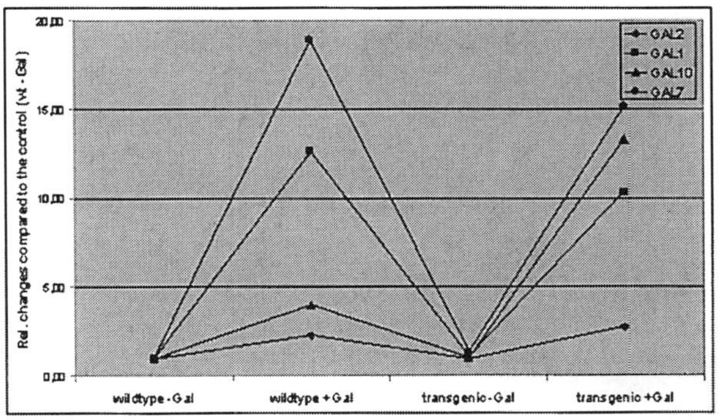

Fig. 3: Transcriptional profile of four yeast genes (see panel) under four growth conditions listed along the x-axis. Complex cDNAs were made from the relevant yeast cultures and hybridised to an array of all about 6,200 yeast genes. Alterations in mRNA levels were up to nearly twenty-fold for the genes shown.

While the comparison of two experimental conditions is relatively simple, although not trivial considering the large number of genes, good data management is essential for such analyses, even if only relatively few experiments are analysed. Also critical is a thorough data assessment, since only good raw data will result in good data interpretation. Last, the extraction of biologically useful information is the most challenging task. Although especially the last issue is far from being developed to any satisfactory status, important analyses are already possible [5]. One of the most critical aspects is the data processing (Fig. 4).

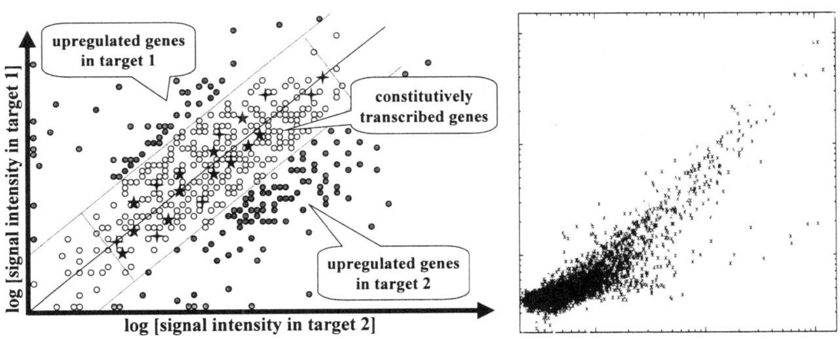

Fig. 4: Scatter plot presentation of transcript profiles. Left, a part of a correlation plot between two experimental data sets is shown. Dots represent relative signal intensities of genes in the two complex hybridisations. Alongside the diagonal are genes expressed at approximately the same levels in both experiments. The barred diagonal lines define the thresholds of significant variation – grey gene spots beyond the threshold lines represent differentially transcribed genes. Data within the rectangle of barred lines have been used for normalisation of both data sets. Alternatively, a set of housekeeping genes (★) or externally added controls (✦) can be used to make both data sets comparable. In the right panel, unprocessed expression data of approximately 6,200 yeast-genes under two different experimental conditions were plotted. The axes represent raw intensity values. The „banana“ shape can be a typical effect prior to background correction.

A complex hybridisation might exhibit an individual background. This can be averaged over the whole filter or individually corrected for each spot. Second, the quality of the target-DNA and many other factors influence the strength of a signal. Thus, correction factors have to be included to make two data sets comparable. Third, thresholds have to be defined, by which a gene is classified as significantly up- or down-regulated. For correction, either the majority of constitutive data, housekeeping genes with a known constitutive expression or external controls added during target generation can be used to normalise two data sets.

Chips and chemistry

For chip-based analyses, the probe is usually attached to glass slides and target-DNAs are labelled with fluorescent dyes (Fig. 5), most commonly Cy3 and Cy5.

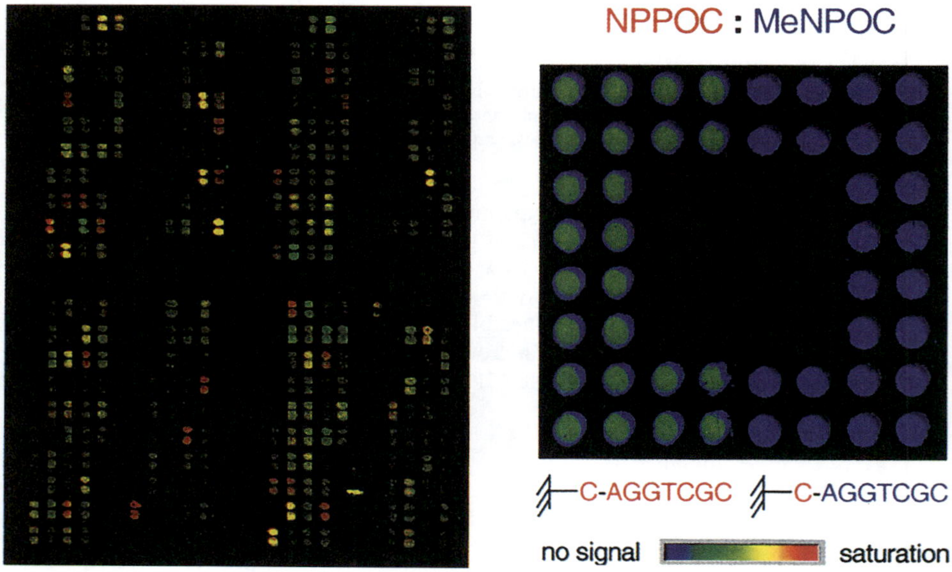

Fig. 5: DNA-microarrays. Left panel: two clone libraries (resulting from RDA experiments) were amplified and PCR products spotted in duplicate on glass slides. Hybridisation of a Cy3- (red) and a Cy5-labelled (green) complex target were performed in parallel. Differentially expressed genes show up in either green or red. Yellow signals indicate an identical amont of the corresponding cDNA being present in both probes. Right panel: comparison of NPPOC and the MeNPOC photochemistry, the latter commercially used by Affymetrix for light-directed DNA-chip synthesis. The more than threefold difference in the synthesis yield was visualised by hybridisation with a complementary, fluorescently labelled oligonucleotide (reproduced with permission from Oxford University Press, ref. [7]).

Because of their different spectrum, two targets can be applied simultaneously. However, glass also has disadvantages. More conventional support media like nylon membranes have a much higher binding capacity for nucleic acids due to their 3-dimensional structure. In addition, more sophisticated technical equipment is required to achieve equal spot qualities on flat surfaces. Furthermore, many glass chips are designed only for single use. In our group, various sorts of microarrays are prepared, from *in situ* synthesised oligomer arrays made of deoxynucleotides or peptide nucleic acids to slides onto which pre-fabricated material such as PCR-products is spotted (Fig. 5). For all applications, basically one chemistry is used [6] (Fig. 6), which attaches the biomolecules covalently to the glass surface. This strategy also permits variation of the loading capacity, charge and hydrophobicity. For the photolithographically controlled *in situ* synthesis of oligonucleotides, a combination of high-yielding photochemistry based on the NPPOCprotection group and an on-line quality control at each individual array position was recently developed [7], resulting in a well-defined system for much improved analysis.

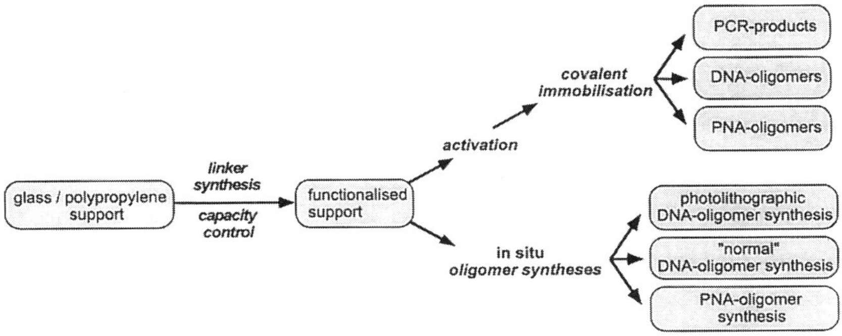

Fig. 6: Variable surface chemistry for covalent attachment of biomolecules. All forms of DNA-arrays currently used in our laboratory can be served with a single linker systems (reproduced with permission from Oxford University Press, ref. [6]).

Substitution of DNA by PNA for mutational analyses

Peptide nucleic acid (PNA) is an alternative class of molecule to be used as a probe in hybridisation experiments [8]. A peptide backbone replaces the sugar-phosphate backbone of nucleic acids. The properties of peptide nucleic acids allow a specific hybridisation to a DNA or RNA target at even higher selectivity. Also, PNA is not degraded by either proteases or nucleases. Last, it is an uncharged molecule. Therefore, no ions are required to counteract interstrand repulsion between probe and target, as is required in case of DNA-probe. One application is the detection of single nucleotide mutations for diagnostic purposes. The region of few bases around a known point mutation is covered by PNA oligomers offset from each other by a single nucleotide, in comparison with the corresponding set of PNA-oligomers covering the wildtype (Fig. 7). DNA is hybridised to this array and allows the detection of homozygous and heterozygous point mutations.

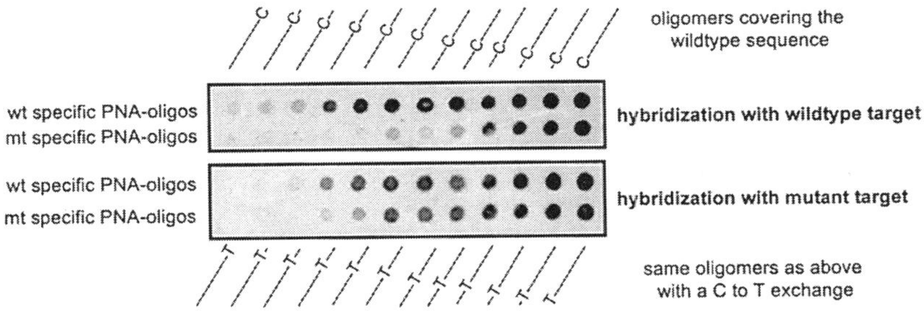

Fig. 7: A known point mutation (a C to T exchange) in a gene responsible for a higher susceptibility for breast cancer was investigated for its occurrence in patient-DNA. Each panel contains an upper lane of PNA oligomer-spots covering the wildtype allele and a bottom lane of the very similar PNA oligomers bearing the mutation. Labelled DNAs of two individual samples were hybridised and showed different signal patterns, exhibiting either only a good binding to the wildtype oligos in the sample of the person with the wildtype allele only, or binding to both oligomer lanes in case of the individual being heterozygous for the mutation.

Outlook

With the advent of several methods for a large scale analysis of genomic and transcriptional information, the understanding of intracellular activities on a molecular level has become within reach, at least at the level of nucleic acids. With further refinements currently under development, RDA should be applicable in near future to comparisons between the transcriptional state of single cells. A major problem will be the choice and generation of the starting material without introducing experimentally caused biases. Transcriptional profiling currently is a technique, which is applied after finishing the sequence analysis of a genome. However, this order could be turned around, first generating profile data and directedly sequencing only those genomic regions that exhibit an interesting functional response.

References

[1] N. Lisitsyn *et al*, Cloning the differences between two complex genomes, *Science* **259** (1993) 946-951.
[2] M. Hubank, and D. G. Schatz, Identifying differences in mRNA expression by representational difference analysis of cDNA, *Nucleic Acids Res.* **22** (1994) 5640-5648.
[3] S. M. Welfort *et al*, Detection of differentially expressed genes in primary tumor tissues using representational differences analysis coupled to microarray hybridization **26** (1998) 3059-3065.
[4] J. D. Hoheisel, Oligomer chip technology. *Trends Biotechnol.* **15** (1997) 465-469.
[5] A. A. Alizadeh *et al*, Distinct types of diffuse large B-cell lymphoma identified by gene expression profiling, *Nature* **403** (2000). 503-511.
[6] M. Beier and J. D. Hoheisel, Versatile derivatisation of solid support media for covalent bonding on DNA-microchips, *Nucleic Acids Res.* **27** (1999) 1970-1977.
[7] M. Beier and J. D. Hoheisel, Production by quantitative photolithographic synthesis of individually quality-checked DNA microarrays, *Nucleic Acids Res.* **28** (2000) e11.
[8] S. Matysiak *et al*, PNA-arrays for nucleic acid detection. In: P. Nielsen and M. Egholm (Eds.), *Peptide Nucleic Acids: Protocols and Applications*, Horizon Scientific Press, Wymondham (1999) pp 119-128.

Molecular Pathogenesis of Pancreatic Cancer
T.M. Gress (Ed.)
IOS Press, 2000

High-throughput Technologies and Resources

John O'Brien, Dolores Cahill, Uwe Radelof, Hans Lehrach
Max-Planck-Institut für Molekulare Genetik, Ihnestraße 73, D-14195 Berlin, Germany
Cornelia Maurer
Resource Centre/Primary Database, Heubnerweg 6, D-14059 Berlin, Germany

Abstract. The role of Hans Lehrach's group in the Pancreatic Cancer consortium is essentially to provide clones and high-density filters to other members of the consortium and also access to the high-throughput technologies developed in the group. A brief description of some of these technologies and their applications is presented here. The Resource Centre/Primary Database (RZPD) of the German Human Genome Project was founded largely from within the group and has played to date the greatest part in providing these facilities to the rest of the consortium. The services and facilities available at the RZPD are also briefly outlined.

1. Robotic Library Picking and Spotting

For many genomic or genetic analyses large libraries in the order of tens of thousands of clones are required. Manual procedures are clearly inadequate for reliable processing of such large numbers of clones. We describe in this section robotic systems to pick libraries from large agar plates and array them into 384-well microtiter plates, and which can then arrange the clones in highly dense grids on nylon membranes or glass slides. Following the development of the first prototypes in Hans Lehrach's group [1], such systems are now being used in a number of laboratories throughout the world.

The picking robots are based on an image analysis program and an array of metal pins which can be moved to any position over a table which holds the agar plates and microtiter plates. The robot photographs an area of the agar plate and identifies the positions of all colonies present. The software then makes judgements concerning the size and roundness of colonies, their separation from each other and their colour (e.g. for blue/white selection), and it can also distinguish air bubbles in the agar. Based on these decisions, a list of the co-ordinates of all suitable colonies in the field of view is drawn up. An actuator, controlling the pin array, is moved into position above each colony in turn and fires out a narrow metal pin into the colony, thereby taking up a small sample of cells. When all the pins (96) have „picked" a colony, the actuator is moved to the rear of the robot where a microtiter plate is inoculated and the array of pins cleaned and sterilised. This cycle repeats until all the identified colonies have been picked, then another section of the agar plate is photographed and the process continues.

The robots can typically pick up to 3,500 colonies per hour, with the only human intervention being, after start-up and calibration, to feed in and remove agar plates and microtiter plates.

After a library has been picked several copies are made and all microtiter plates are bar-coded with the library name, copy number and plate number. The original copy, or master copy, is stored separately to safeguard against loss of the library due to power cuts etc. and the others are used as working copies.

The other major robotic system for library handling is the gridding or spotting robot. This consists of a table where up to 24 nylon membranes or 180 glass slides are spread out, and a stacker which holds the library copy to be spotted. A robotic arm removes a microtiter plate from the stacker and places it in a holder. Here the lid is removed and the bar-code is read. A spotting „gadget", an array of 384 metal pins, then comes into position above the plate such that each pin is aligned with a microtiter plate well. The pins dip into the wells, each one taking a very small droplet (c. 4 nL) away with them.

The gadget then moves into position above the membrane (or slide) and moves down until the pins touch the membrane's surface. When the gadget withdraws, the droplet remains on the membrane. This step is then repeated for each membrane on the robot table, then the microtiter plate lid is replaced, the plate returned to the stacker, the gadget is sterilised and dried and the next plate is taken from the stacker.

By using very small offsets, a high density of spots can be achieved. Although higher densities are achievable we routinely use c. 125 spots/cm^2, which translates to 57,600 spots on a 22cm x 22cm membrane. Typically the clones are spotted in duplicate along with guide spots and control clones, which reduces the figure to a little more than 25,000 clones per membrane but the gain in reliability and accuracy of spot identification more than justifies this.

The spotting robots are most often used with bacterial cultures, in which case the membrane is removed from the robot table, placed on an agar plate and incubated overnight. After the colonies have grown the membranes are then processed to lyse the cells, denature and fix the DNA and wash away the cell debris. The membrane is then ready for use in mapping projects, gene searches, library characterisation, complex hybridisations, and other uses.

2. Oligonucleotide Fingerprinting

To effectively characterise a cDNA library it is necessary to know how many different genes are represented, it is often useful to know how many copies of each gene are present, and it is desirable to be able to say which of those genes are previously known. The technique oligonucleotide fingerprinting [2-4] is a means of answering these questions.

The essence of the technique is that a PCR copy of the library is made and spotted onto nylon membranes as described above. These membranes thus carry only the cDNA inserts of each clone and no *E. coli* or vector DNA. They are then hybridised with a series of 200 radio-labelled oligonucleotides (8mers). After each hybridisation the positive signals are visualised using phosphor storage screens. The images from these are analysed using software designed in the department for this purpose. An intensity value is calculated for each clone and stored. After all 200 hybridisations are complete a fingerprint, a list of the signals obtained for each oligonucleotide, is constructed for each clone. This fingerprint is characteristic of the clone's DNA sequence and can therefore be used to group related clones together into clusters, with each cluster representing a gene.

In this way the number of genes represented in the library can be determined and, for each gene, an indication of its level of expression is given by the size of the cluster. Furthermore, using the known DNA sequences of the 200 oligonucleotides, theoretical fingerprints can be constructed for all expressed sequences in a database such as GenBank.

By comparison with the experimental fingerprints, many genes can be assigned an identity and candidate novel genes are pinpointed.

The oligofingerprinting technique is therefore a rapid method of characterising a large library. As different membranes can be hybridised simultaneously to the same oligonucleotide, we have been able to efficiently analyse libraries of 100,000 clones, from PCR to clustering, in a time period of four months. The technique can also be applied to reduce redundancy in large-scale shotgun sequencing projects [3].

3. Complex Hybridisations

There are currently several groups assembling large non-redundant sets of human genes*. The main goal of these projects is to make a defined set of clones for use in complex hybridisations, where a (complex) mixture of mRNA species isolated from a tissue or cell type is hybridised against an array of these clones. The signal from each spot in the array depends on the amount of the corresponding mRNA species in the probe and so the activity of each gene in the original tissue or cell type can be measured.

In collaboration with the group of Annemarie Poustka in the Deutsche Krebsforschungszentrum (DKFZ), the department and the RZPD have produced an arrayed set of 36,000 PCR products, each one representing a different gene. This set has been produced by clustering the NCBI human EST database and choosing a representative from each cluster according to several stringent criteria (e.g. length of clone, quality of sequence data, number of reads available). We have arrayed these PCR products onto glass slides and are developing techniques for two-colour hybridisations, adapting our existing image analysis software for this purpose. In parallel, the identity of all genes in the set is being verified by oligofingerprinting and sequencing.

Using this large, well characterised, non-redundant set, we are applying existing techniques and procedures still under development to perform complex hybridisations quickly and reliably. This will form the basis of a high-throughput approach, where many samples can be hybridised in parallel to these arrays. This approach will be particularly useful for the study of disease states by comparing mRNA samples from diseased tissues with samples from the corresponding healthy tissues.

4. Protein Arrays

Transcriptional activity is only one aspect of the overall state of a tissue or cell type. Of more fundamental relevance is the analysis of the proteins present. It is possible to use the robotic systems described above to also array expression libraries and to process the membranes in such a way that the expressed proteins are bound to the filters and the rest of the cell material is washed away [5]. This technology is already in place, using a modified cDNA cloning vector to ensure that transcription can occur in all three possible reading frames, and to increase protein yield. Also a tag is introduced so that false positives (short peptides expressed from incorrect reading frames) can be eliminated.

Such protein arrays can be used to link data from DNA studies with data from protein studies - for example, if a cDNA library is analysed by oligonucleotide fingerprinting, the same library can be arrayed as expressed proteins and data from the cDNA clones linked

---

* http://www.ncbi.nlm.nih.gov/UniGene/index.html
http://www.genomesystems.com/expression/clonelists/index.html
http://www.resgen.com/products/AFFYEXP_protocol_pf.php3

to data from the proteins. The subset of the library which gives positive signals for the tag can be re-arrayed with reference to the oligofingerprinting data to form a non-redundant protein expression sublibrary, which in the form of a micro-array (see below), could be applied to characterising antibody binding specificity, screening the protein array with peptides to discover what proteins such peptides bind, profiling of sera from normal versus disease patients, and screening for protein-protein or ligand-receptor interactions [6].

5. Other Technologies

To date, the classical two-hybrid system for the identification of protein-protein interactions is applied only at laboratory scale, where the single steps of the procedure are serial, time-consuming and not appropriate for the analysis of large numbers of probes. In the standard two-hybrid system only one bait protein is used for screening for novel interacting partner proteins. The group of Erich Wanker has used complete genetic libraries for the synthesis of "fish" proteins as well as of bait proteins. Such a system could be applied to generate a network of protein-protein interactions on a large scale. For this purpose, additional selection procedures were combined with modern automation techniques. Using this system, a huntingtin interacting protein (HIP1), which is a novel protein with significant homology to the yeast protein Sla2, has been identified [7].

To study developmental stages in model organisms, such as sea urchin, zebrafish and amphioxus, we have developed a high-throughput *in situ* hybridisation pipeline. For example in the zebrafish project interesting cDNA clones, as determined by oligonucleotide fingerprinting, are hybridised to zebrafish embryos, from various developmental stages, to determine their expression patterns. In collaboration with Dr. Bernhard Hermann of the MPI for Immunobiology we have a similar project with mouse embryos. In this way we aim to correlate gene activity across developmental stages and across species and phyla.

Several groups have made use of the high-throughput techniques in mapping projects. For example large sequence-ready contigs (> 3Mb) from human chromosome 21 have been constructed using high-throughput non-radioactive hybridisations to cosmid and PAC libraries [8]. Also a mapping project in mouse has incorporated four different YAC libraries into a single map by using interspersed repetitive sequences as hybridisation probes [9]. This project has relied heavily on the robotic systems and high-throughput hybridisation technologies described here, to characterise 600 individual probes per week against the full set of 75,000 YAC clones.

The robotic systems used in these projects are themselves undergoing improvements, with particular emphasis on miniaturisation. Already, dense „micro-arrays“ are being produced on glass slides for complex hybridisations, and also a robotic system that automates all the steps in a hybridisation has been built. Piezoelectric dispensers are being developed for very low volume, rapid micro-arraying which is particularly suitable for preparing MALDI-MS targets and there is a project to convert oligonucleotide fingerprinting to a mass spectrometry based procedure, which will greatly improve the rapidity and discrimination.

All of the technologies and projects mentioned here have relied heavily on database and analysis software written in the department. Analysis of the hybridisation images is conducted by Unix-based programs which first identify every spot in the array and then assigns each one an intensity. The program is very flexible with regard to size and geometry of the array and also internal order (or spotting pattern) of clones. Clustering software for the oligonucleotide fingerprinting has also been written within the group [10] as well as mapping programs for assembling hybridisation data [11,12]. Both within the Max-Planck-Institute and the RZPD, databases are of crucial importance and a lot of work has been done to develop appropriate tools for our own databases and for querying and integrating with external databases [13].

6. Facilities of the RZPD

As the central infrastructure unit of the German Human Genome Project the Resource Centre has been funded by the Federal Ministry of Education and Research (BMBF) since 1995. It is jointly operated by the Max-Planck-Institute for Molecular Genetics (Dept. Hans Lehrach) in Berlin and the Deutsches Krebsforschungszentrum (Dept. Annemarie Poustka) in Heidelberg.

The Resource Centre has one of the most comprehensive collections of genomic and cDNA gene libraries of man, as well as of selected model organisms, world-wide and offers its customers a wide product range for the libraries in question This offer comprises high-density clone filters, protein and DNA-filters, clone and DNA pools or individual clones of the different libraries but also includes a great variety of services. By means of the UniGene sets of man, mouse, rat, zebrafish and arabidopsis the RZPD are in a position to provide the scientific community with one of the largest collections of non-redundant EST sets. The size of these "UniGene Sets" is constantly enlarged by collaboration and self-production. Furthermore, the Resource Centre is one of only 5 authorised distributors of I.M.A.G.E. ESTs which is, with more than 1,3 million clones, the greatest public EST-collection currently available.

The RZPD already has 6 pancreatic cDNA libraries, as well as the 6 pancreatic or pancreatic tumour libraries contained within the IMAGE collection, available. These libraries are available as colony filters, as individual clones or as pools. In addition to this, the Resource Centre offers as a service, the possibility to generate, pick, spot and array, custom made libraries.

As mentioned above, the Resource Centre lays particular emphasis on collating all clone-related experimental data (sequence, mapping, expression, *in situ* hybridisation) into the primary database. This data can be retrieved through the world wide web, in user friendly graphical interfaces where appropriate. In addition to a wide range of predefined standard query forms which are already in place, user-defined queries are currently being enabled for maximum flexibility.

All materials and services provided by the Resource Centre are available not only to the groups engaged in the German Human Genome Project but also to all scientists from research and industry at home and abroad. Nearly 5,000 registered users and a constantly increasing demand for the research tools offered clearly prove the success of this facility. Further information is available through its website - http://www.rzpd.de/.

7. Summary

The techniques and facilities described here are all based on the idea that experiments in molecular biology are most effectively performed massively parallel and in high-throughput. By screening large libraries, the chance of finding positive signals is greatly increased, and by testing many samples in parallel experiments, the amount of data obtained is maximised.

The associated idea is to join the various techniques into a pipeline to link data from diverse sources together. For example, a cDNA library from an interesting disease tissue is fingerprinted to determine what genes are present, and any novel genes are sequenced. Interesting clones are used as probes for whole-mount *in situ* hybridisations to several tissue samples, to monitor expression of the genes at different stages of the disease. Based on the patterns obtained some clones are expressed as proteins and used to „fish" a yeast 2-hybrid library to find interacting proteins, which can in turn be used to screen antibody libraries. From this experiment antibody probes for further investigations are found and all of these data are combined together in a unified database.

The combination of this approach with the many libraries and other facilities available at the RZPD is a powerful tool for any biological investigation. Together with clinical and epidemiological data, information about active genes, sequence data, transcription and translation levels, spatial and temporal gene expression patterns, interacting proteins and analogues in other species can be brought together to form a comprehensive and detailed picture of the progress of a disease.

References

[1] S. Meier-Ewert, *et al.*, An automated approach to generating expressed sequence catalogues, *Nature* **361** (1993) 375-376.

[2] S. Meier-Ewert, *et al.*, Comparative gene expression profiling by oligonucleotide fingerprinting, *Nucleic Acids Research* **26** (1998) 2216-2223.

[3] U. Radelof, *et al.*, Preselection of shotgun clones by oligonucleotide fingerprinting: an efficient and high throughput strategy to reduce redundancy in large-scale sequencing projects, *Nucleic Acids Research* **26** (1998) 5358-5364.

[4] A. J. Poustka, *et al.*, Toward the gene catalogue of sea urchin development: the construction and analysis of an unfertilized egg cDNA library highly normalized by oligonucleotide fingerprinting, *Genomics* **59** (1999) 122-133.

[5] K. Bussow, *et al.*, A method for global protein expression and antibody screening on high-density filters of an arrayed cDNA library, *Nucleic Acids Research* **26** (1998) 5007-5008.

[6] A. Lueking, *et al.*, Protein microarrays for gene expression and antibody screening, *Analytical Biochemistry* **270** (1999) 103-111.

[7] E. E. Wanker, *et al.*, HIP-I: a huntingtin interacting protein isolated by the yeast two-hybrid system, *Human Molecular Genetics* **6** (1997) 487-495.

[8] T. Hildmann, *et al.*, A contiguous 3-Mb sequence-ready map in the S3-MX region on 21q22.2 based on high- throughput nonisotopic library screenings, *Genome Research* **9** (1999) 360-372.

[9] K. W. Hunter, *et al.*, Toward the construction of integrated physical and genetic maps of the mouse genome using interspersed repetitive sequence PCR (IRS-PCR) genomics, *Genome Research* **6** (1996) 290-299.

[10] R. Herwig, *et al.*, Large-Scale Clutering of cDNA-Fingerprinting Data, *Genome Research* **9** (1999) 1093-1105.

[11] R. Mott, *et al.*, Algorithms and software tools for ordering clone libraries: application to the mapping of the genome of Schizosaccharomyces pombe, *Nucleic Acids Research* **21** (1993) 1965-1974.

[12] A. Grigoriev, A. Levin, and H. Lehrach, A distributed environment for physical map construction, *Bioinformatics* **14** (1998) 252-258.

[13] S. Schulze-Kremer, Adding semantics to genome databases: towards an ontology for molecular biology, *ISMB* **5** (1997) 272-275.

Author Index